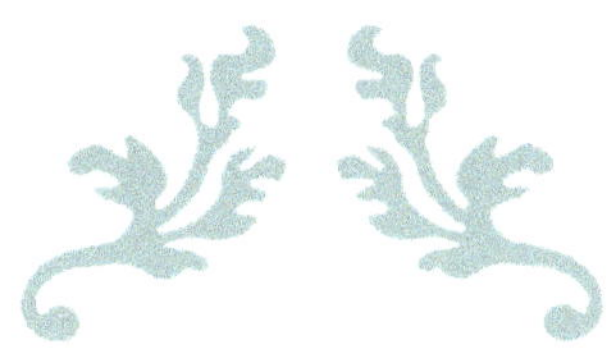

Confronting the Cancer Care Plight:

Using First Principles to Navigate Your Cancer Journey

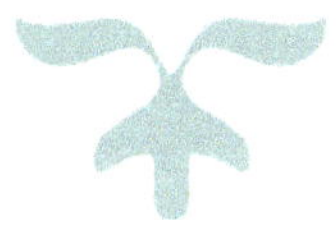

XUEWU LIU

Xuewu Liu

Beijing, China

liuxuewu@wanbincell.com

myxcancer.com

From Idea to Print: The Birth of This Book

Whether you are a patient newly diagnosed with cancer, a long-term survivor, or a family member or friend of someone with cancer, you will inevitably delve into the current state of cancer care. You may believe that you have chosen the best treatment option available, but you are likely unsatisfied with the outcomes and yearn for better solutions.

I initially ventured into the field of biology, driven by a commitment to seek improved treatment options for cancer patients I knew. My non-medical background, coupled with extensive experience in the complex fields of atmospheric science and economics, enabled me to develop a straightforward and practical framework for tackling complex scientific challenges during the process of developing a new drug that aligns with the long-term interests of cancer patients. This framework coincidentally aligns with the innovative thinking behind SpaceX's development of groundbreaking reusable rockets.

The complexity of cancer treatment far exceeds that of rocket launches, not because the technology required is more complex, but due to the inherent intricacies of the cancer treatment process itself. However, the paradigm shifts in breaking conventional thinking are remarkably similar in both fields.

In economics, there is a fundamental principle that the provision of public goods is inefficient in the absence of direct involvement by stakeholders. Before Elon Musk founded SpaceX, national space launch services were such public goods. The introduction of profit-motivated companies into the space launch market led to a transformative shift in thinking and the emergence of reusable rocket technology.

In the realm of cancer care, I have observed that patient involvement is minimal, which may be a contributing factor to the globally low quality of cancer treatment. Drawing a parallel, just as Musk applied first principles to achieve cost-effective space launches, allowing SpaceX to dominate 90% of the global space launch market, similar innovative thinking could revolutionize cancer treatment standards.

This book, "Confronting the Cancer Care Plight: Using First Principles to Navigate Your Cancer Journey," is crafted against this backdrop. It encourages cancer patients to actively participate in their treatment process and provides a set of principles based on first principles thinking to help patients achieve the true goal of cancer treatment: to live a high-quality life while effectively combating the disease.

This book was completed in April 2024.

Table of Contents

PREFACE

As we journey through life, the specter of cancer looms large, presenting a formidable challenge that many of us may eventually face. When confronted with cancer, our priorities shift dramatically, with life itself swiftly rising to the forefront of our concerns, relegating all else to the background. Our immediate focus narrows to combating this disease. While many adhere strictly to their doctor's recommendations, selecting treatments reputed for their efficacy and cost-effectiveness, this path is not the sole option. It is crucial to recognize that, although contemporary cancer treatments might appear limited, this does not necessarily reflect on the reliability of medical advice. On the contrary, I believe the reason for the inadequacy in cancer treatment levels is that the entire cancer treatment system does not aim to address the fundamental issues of cancer.

Globally, the data reveals a startling uniformity in cancer treatment technologies across various age groups and nations, suggesting that advancements in systems, economies, and technologies have not significantly enhanced the value delivered to cancer patients. Moreover, there is a pervasive trend of overtreatment within the healthcare system dedicated to cancer care. Standardized clinical guidelines, while providing uniform treatment options, restrict the choices available to both physicians and patients, diminishing the patients' involvement in their own treatment decisions. Consequently, the treatment plans prescribed, though based on these guidelines, may not always align with the patients' long-term interests, particularly in terms of sustaining a quality life. Furthermore, the emphasis on early detection and treatment can also act as a catalyst for overtreatment.

Facing the cancer care plight, as a cancer patient, wouldn't you want to reclaim your voice and break free from this predicament?

Inspired by SpaceX's revolutionary approach to rocket launch technology, which utilizes reusable components for enhanced cost-effectiveness, we can adopt a similar mindset in cancer care. This approach, known as first principles thinking, championed by Elon Musk, challenges us to discard conventional dependencies on analogies, precedents, and conventional wisdom. Instead, it involves deconstructing complex concepts, problems, or beliefs to their most fundamental components and rigorously examining the core of the issues.

Our lives are governed by various principles, shaped by our values, perceptions, belief systems, and reasoning methods. These principles influence our opinions and allow our brains to employ previously learned conclusions as shortcuts in thinking. Often, we adhere to these principles without questioning their foundational assumptions. While these principles may have been valid at their inception, questioning their relevance today necessitates that we overturn outdated theories and forge new realities for ourselves.

First principles thinking encourages us to embrace a new mindset, recognizing when traditional methods become obsolete. This shift in thinking eschews conventional wisdom, cuts through dogma, and challenges our own beliefs. While first principles thinking and traditional reductionism both emphasize deconstructing problems into their elemental parts, they differ in their applications and impacts. First principles thinking focuses on controlled, thoughtful examination at a foundational level, whereas reductionism often reduces problems to a microscopic scale. This distinction allows first principles thinking to provide more profound and innovative solutions to complex issues like cancer treatment, enabling us not only to better understand the nature of cancer but potentially to uncover more effective treatments.

In the realm of modern medicine, which often remains entrenched in a reductionist approach, applying first principles thinking is crucial. For cancer, this means thinking at the cellular rather than the molecular level, which is often the focus of cutting-edge research in molecular biology or genetics. By reevaluating the causes and processes of cancer through first principles and developing treatment strategies at the cellular level, we can utilize mathematical models to ensure logical completeness and accuracy, provided the input data and model settings are correct.

In this book, I introduce a life model that simplifies life into a mathematical framework, helping us pinpoint the primary factors and processes impacting life. By applying the life model, we can perceive cancer as a manifestation of aging, encapsulating the essence and treatment methods of the disease. I believe the life model exemplifies a precise application of first principles in disease management.

We address cancer using a first principles approach, following a structured process: identifying the issue, breaking it down, analyzing its fundamental components, reassembling the information, and using life models as tools for reasoning. We've further developed a cancer model consistent with these principles, leading us to the best strategies for combating cancer—a comprehensive framework for evaluating cancer therapies. Our optimal cancer treatment plan includes combinations or legal variations of approved therapies, in compliance with existing medical regulations. We discuss experimental treatments only in the context of potential future advancements in cancer care. Through this book, I aim to encourage cancer patients to actively engage in their treatment decisions and assist them in making the best choices under current conditions.

PART ONE: FIRST PRINCIPLES IN CANCER TREATMENT

"We are enjoying longer and healthier lives than ever before, until the moment cancer strikes."

"SpaceX is using first principles to lower costs to launch rockets into space with the end goal of making human life multi-planetary. "

1. CANCER TREATMENT LIMITATIONS: SIGNIFICANT PLIGHT IMPACTING PATIENT CARE

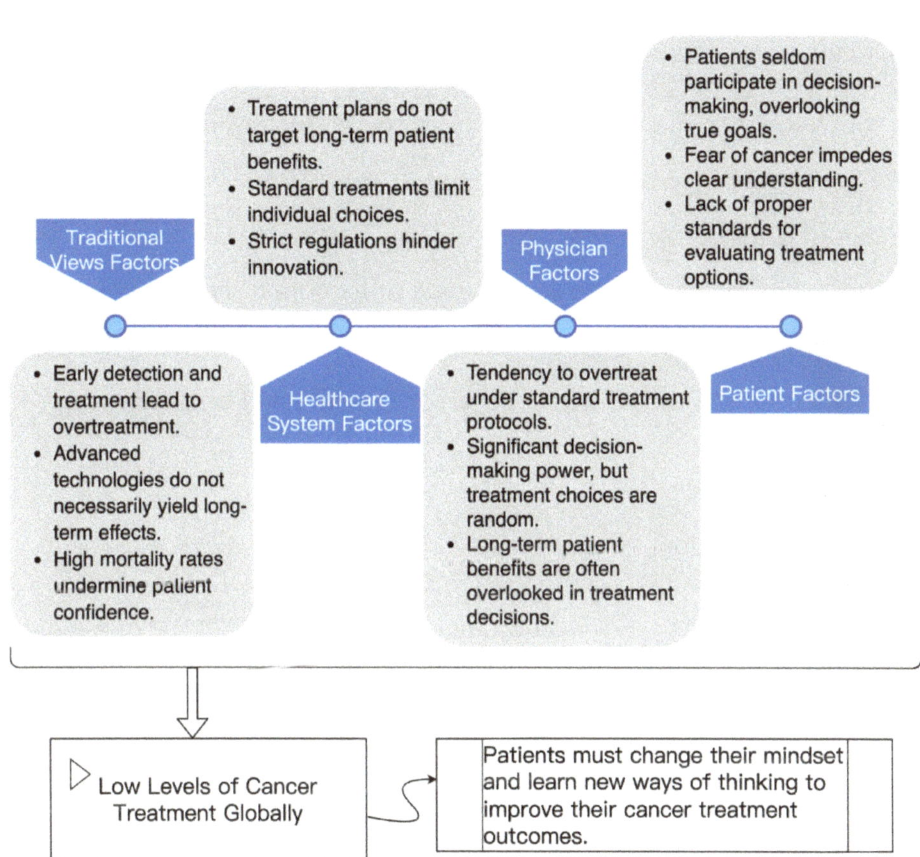

Living long enough almost inevitably brings you face-to-face with cancer, with the lifetime risk of developing it nearing 20%. This certainly makes cancer seem like a common occurrence. However, once diagnosed, many people feel the looming shadow of death, filled with fear and anxiety. At this point, you might find yourself focusing solely on treatment, with everything else taking a backseat.

In such circumstances, choosing the right doctor and treatment plan becomes crucial. You have the option to passively follow your doctor's recommendations or actively seek out the treatment you believe is most suitable. Understanding the current state of modern cancer treatments can help you make more informed decisions and find a treatment plan that is both scientifically sound and tailored to your personal situation.

1.1 Global Cancer Data

In 2022, nearly 20 million new cases of cancer were reported worldwide, with 9.7 million people dying from the disease. Looking at data from the United States, there has been a noticeable decline in cancer mortality over the past 20 years, suggesting significant advancements in American cancer treatment technologies. However, a different perspective might reveal a less optimistic situation.

For example, in 1999, 560,000 people died from cancer in the U.S., with a death rate of 201 per 100,000 people. By 2022, the number of deaths had increased to 600,000, but the death rate per 100,000 people had dropped to 181, indicating only a 10% decrease in the mortality rate. This suggests that despite technological progress, the actual impact on extending the lives of cancer patients may not be as significant as hoped.

Moreover, while the U.S. is often seen as a leader in cancer treatment, its cancer mortality rate does not stand out significantly on the global stage. U.S. cancer mortality rates are lower than some developed countries but are comparable to China's and higher than those of Brazil, India, and Indonesia—three developing nations. After adjusting for age, the cancer mortality rates in most countries worldwide typically range from 80 to 100 per 100,000 people, with only minor differences between countries, except for India, which is slightly lower.

These statistics indicate that despite substantial investments in cancer treatment, the U.S. has not achieved a correspondingly low mortality rate. This may mean that compared to some developing countries with less advanced medical conditions, U.S. cancer treatment technologies do not have a significant advantage. This situation reflects a common challenge in the global field of cancer treatment: how to more effectively utilize existing resources and technologies to truly improve the survival rates and quality of life for cancer patients.

Countries or Regions	Mortality (per 100,000 population)	Age-Standardized Mortality Rate	Incidence Age-Standardized Rate
United States	180.9	82.3	367
European Union	236.4	106.5	268.1
United Kingdom	265.4	98.3	307.8
Germany	301.8	99.7	274.2

France	290.6	106.7	339
Japan	339.4	78.6	267.1
China	182.3	96.5	201.6
Brazil	129.5	91.3	214.4
Indonesia	87	82.5	136.9
India	65.2	64.4	98.5

In the United States, despite the continuous introduction of hundreds of new cancer drugs, the real-world effectiveness and impact on patients' quality of life remain significant concerns. Many new drugs are approved on the basis that they can extend a patient's life by a few months. However, this extension often comes at the cost of reducing the quality of life.

For cancer patients in the U.S., even with access to advanced medical care, substantial health insurance, and the latest anti-cancer drugs and technologies, their survival time may not be longer than that of patients in China who are treated with the most cost-effective medications. Intriguingly, some cancer patients in China who choose to forego any treatment might experience longer survival times and higher quality of life.

This indicates that cancer treatment is not just a matter of medical technology but involves a complex decision-making process that considers treatment effectiveness, economic burden, and quality of life. For cancer patients and their families, the choice of treatment should not solely focus on the sophistication of the technology but should also consider the real impact of the treatment on quality of life.

1.2 Current Cancer Treatment Methods

When a cancer patient visits a hospital, the doctor will offer the following treatment options:

Surgery: The goal of surgery is to remove as much of the cancer as possible. This includes procedures like lumpectomy for breast cancer, prostatectomy for prostate cancer, and colectomy for colon cancer.

Interventional Therapy: Similar to surgery, interventional therapy uses specialized instruments inserted directly into the tumor to kill cancer cells on-site through physical or chemical means. Techniques include radiofrequency ablation and photodynamic therapy.

Chemotherapy: This treatment employs drugs to kill cancer cells, with common options including paclitaxel, cisplatin, doxorubicin, and methotrexate.

Radiation Therapy: This method uses high-energy beams, such as X-rays and protons, to destroy cancer cells. It can be delivered externally (external beam radiation) or internally (brachytherapy), with applications like external beam radiation for lung cancer, brachytherapy for cervical cancer, and proton therapy for brain tumors.

Bone Marrow Transplant: Also known as stem cell transplant, this procedure uses your own or donor cells to replace bone marrow and produce new blood cells. It allows for higher doses of chemotherapy and replaces diseased marrow.

Immunotherapy: Also referred to as biological therapy, this approach boosts the immune system's ability to recognize and attack cancer cells. Drugs such as pembrolizumab, nivolumab, ipilimumab, and atezolizumab are used to enhance this response.

Hormone Therapy: Used for hormone-driven cancers like breast and prostate cancer, this therapy removes or blocks hormones that promote cancer growth. Examples include tamoxifen for breast cancer and leuprolide for prostate cancer.

Targeted Drug Therapy: This treatment focuses on specific abnormalities within cancer cells that sustain them. Examples include trastuzumab for HER2-positive breast cancer and imatinib for chronic myeloid leukemia.

With hundreds of cancer treatment methods available, theoretically, there is always one that might suit you, but sometimes having too many options can feel overwhelming.

1.3 Decision Paralysis Caused by Healthcare Systems and Medical Research

The medical system is a strictly regulated field where doctors must adhere to established medical guidelines when communicating with patients. This means that their freedom in offering treatment suggestions is somewhat limited. For cancer patients, doctors' recommendations are usually based on a series of clinical guidelines that provide various diagnostic and treatment options for each type of cancer. Despite this, due to the strict regulation of the industry, the treatment plans doctors propose are often approved therapies, which may not always be in the best interest of the patient. Sometimes, doctors might choose a therapy based on habit or at random, rather than what is most suitable for the patient.

Additionally, medical research is often influenced by reductionism, focusing on sub-cellular or even molecular levels. With technological advancements, humans can now directly observe and manipulate molecules and genes, but this deep dive into research does not always translate into effective treatment methods. In fact, many medical research outcomes, despite being theoretically advanced, have little practical application. For example, although molecular biologists may have identified key genes involved in certain cancers, few new drugs have been developed based on these findings. Instead, many effective new drugs are discovered by chance, suggesting that current cancer research may not always be moving in the right direction.

Recent studies show that new cancer drugs approved in the United States only extend a patient's life by an average of about 2.8 months. This is far too short for cancer patients. In the development process of cancer treatments, researchers and doctors often focus only on whether the treatment can extend life or reduce tumor size, neglecting the impact on the patient's quality of life or the limitations it places on future treatment options. For instance, a new drug might extend a patient's life by three months, but during those months, the patient's quality of life might significantly decline; or after a tumor is surgically removed, continued chemotherapy and radiation to eliminate any remaining cancer cells not only cause long-term side effects but may also damage the patient's immune system and increase the risk of cancer recurrence.

Faced with numerous treatment options, patients and doctors stand at a crossroads with thousands of paths to choose from, each seemingly leading to similar outcomes. This situation can easily lead to decision paralysis, making it difficult to choose the best treatment plan.

1.4 The Chaos of Overtreatment

In China, there is a saying: "Of those who die from cancer, one-third are scared to death, one-third are treated to death, and only the remaining third actually die from the cancer itself." This proverb highlights the dangers of overtreatment.

Currently, clinical cancer treatment relies heavily on three pillars: cancer staging, standardized treatment, and evidence-based medicine. These collectively form the entire cancer treatment system. Cancer staging is used to determine the severity of each patient's condition and to design a "standard treatment" plan for each stage. These treatment plans are based on the results of evidence-based medicine, verified through clinical trials to assess the effectiveness of a treatment method on a group of patients. If a treatment method proves effective or superior for a specific stage in trials, it is recommended for other patients with the same stage. These recommended protocols are submitted to the medical field in the form of expert consensus, known as guidelines. Once published, every doctor is expected to follow the treatment plans described in these guidelines, down to every detail.

However, the reality is that even patients with the same stage of cancer do not always achieve similar results after receiving the same guideline-based treatment. Doctors often attribute these differences to individual variability. This raises a question: knowing that patients differ, why use the same treatment plan for all? Currently, there is no satisfactory explanation. Logically, it doesn't make sense to subject hundreds of thousands of patients to the same treatment plan when many other options are available, as most may not benefit from it.

The full name of the "guidelines" is the "NCCN Clinical Practice Guidelines in Oncology," written and published by the National Comprehensive Cancer Network (NCCN) and updated annually. These guidelines specify detailed treatment methods for each type of cancer and aim to standardize and regulate cancer treatment to improve outcomes and quality. The intent behind the guidelines was to address the chaos in cancer treatment, primarily due to its challenging nature. Given the stakes, it was believed that treatment should be determined by recognized authorities, not left to the discretion of general practitioners. Thus, these guiding documents were created from the collective wisdom and judgment of the most authoritative experts.

Initially, tumor assessment involved merely measuring the size of the primary tumor. It was later found that the number and location of metastases were more crucial for prognosis. Even a small primary tumor can be classified as stage IV if there are multiple distant metastases, indicating a bleak prognosis. Although the primary tumor might be easily removable, guidelines often prohibit surgery if distant metastases are present. However, extensive clinical observations have shown that not all stage IV cancer patients are incurable by surgery; some can be cured. The dilemma is that some people are saved by surgery, while others fare worse, with shortened survival times. Doctors are unclear who will benefit from surgery and who will suffer, so avoiding surgery for all stage IV patients might seem the safest approach. Similarly, outcomes can vary for early-stage patients after the removal of the primary tumor. Although most are cured by surgery, a significant number (10-50%) experience relapse and die.

Once diagnosed with cancer, patients enter a "conveyor belt" of treatment guided by these guidelines. First, the stage of cancer is determined based on tumor size and distribution. If it is early-stage and operable, surgery is performed first, with recurrence dealt with later. For late-stage patients who cannot undergo surgery, radiation, chemotherapy, or targeted therapy is administered until options are exhausted. This "conveyor belt" approach has been in place for decades, based on the logic of evidence-based medicine, which includes: (1) Selecting the best treatment option from past similar cases; (2) Continuing a treatment as long as it works, until it fails; (3) Avoiding unproven treatments. This approach inevitably harms some patients, even if the chosen treatment has a relatively high success rate, as a significant portion may not benefit.

As treatment guidelines have become widespread, the overall level of cancer treatment has improved in the short term due to greater uniformity. However, in the long run, these standardized guidelines have not significantly enhanced treatment levels. Instead, they have simplified cancer treatment to some extent. While standardization has reduced errors and benefited some patients, it has also harmed those not suited for guideline-based treatment.

For example, guidelines might recommend a specific chemotherapy drug as first-line treatment for a certain tumor. Clinical trial data show that this drug is effective for about 70% of patients, which seems reasonable. But why force the remaining 30% to undergo this treatment? The only reason is the lack of alternatives. Because it is impossible to know in advance whether the drug will work for a specific individual, it must be tried to find out. In reality, the greatest benefit of following guidelines is not patient welfare but protection for doctors: even if the world's most authoritative treatment fails, the doctor cannot be blamed.

In today's increasingly tense doctor-patient environment, doctors strictly adhere to guidelines partly to avoid liability. Even high-ranking officials and celebrities may only receive standard treatment because doctors prefer to follow guidelines to reduce liability risks. In such cases, patient outcomes are often less than ideal.

For cancer treatment, both doctors and patients tend to choose the newest, most expensive methods, believing them to be the most effective. However, the approval of new therapies or drugs is often based only on short-term effects in a selected group of people. Therefore, cancer patients should carefully consider the long-term effectiveness and suitability of treatments.

1.5 Debunking the Myth of "Early Detection, Early Treatment" in Cancer

In the medical field, the widely accepted notion is that early detection of cancer is often considered key to improving cure rates and survival. The National Comprehensive Cancer Network (NCCN) vigorously promotes the concept of early cancer screening and treatment. This organization provides up-to-date guidelines for cancer diagnosis and treatment, aimed at helping doctors and patients detect and treat cancer earlier to enhance treatment outcomes and survival rates. Indeed, for cancers like breast cancer and skin cancer, early detection and treatment often lead to better treatment outcomes and relatively higher survival rates. This is because cancer is generally easier to manage in its early stages, and the treatment methods are relatively simpler.

However, this widespread promotion of early screening and treatment also brings some problems, particularly the issues of overdiagnosis and overtreatment. Overdiagnosis refers to the detection through screening of cancers that would not impact the patient's health or lifespan even if left untreated. These cancers may never show any symptoms and might not become life-threatening. However, once diagnosed, patients and doctors usually opt for treatment, leading to the problem of overtreatment.

Overtreatment means aggressively treating these essentially non-dangerous cancers with surgery, radiation, chemotherapy, and other methods, which can themselves cause severe side effects and complications. For example, chemotherapy can lead to nausea, hair loss, and suppression of the immune system, while surgery can cause infections and long-term pain. Additionally, the mental stress, time commitment, and financial burden of treatment are significant burdens that patients must bear.

Overtreatment is one issue, but a bigger problem is that the logic of improving patient survival through early detection and treatment does not always hold up, especially when cancer treatment methods generally have low efficacy. It may only increase the survival period during the early detection and treatment phase, with almost no difference in overall quality of life and final outcomes for the patient. When examining existing cancer treatments, there are virtually no therapies without side effects.

If a cancer patient recovers after treatment, it is impossible to prove that they would not have recovered without treatment; it is generally assumed that it was because the cancer was detected relatively early. If a cancer patient does not respond to treatment, even if the cancer was detected when it was very small, it is often assumed that it was not detected early enough; in medical practice, it is also not feasible to divide cancer patients into groups for controlled studies of treated versus untreated. However, we can still gain considerable insights through the following three approaches.

   <u>Analyzing the impact of early detection, diagnosis, and treatment on cancer outcomes involves looking at changes in cancer incidence, 5-year survival rates, and mortality in a country or region, especially before and after emphasizing these early interventions.</u>

One clinical investigation that highlights this issue began in 1993 in South Korea, where thyroid ultrasound screenings became widespread among the healthy population. This led to a fifteenfold increase in diagnosed thyroid cancer cases by 2011. Regions that conducted more screenings also diagnosed more thyroid cancer cases. However, despite this sharp increase in diagnoses, the mortality rate from thyroid cancer remained unchanged over these 18 years, sparking widespread attention and discussion.

Additionally, a comparative analysis of cancer statistics between the United States and China reveals intriguing phenomena and provides insights. In 2014, major Chinese media outlets reported a striking statistic on the front pages: the 5-year survival rate for cancer in the U.S. was 68%, while in China, it was only 31%. Many naturally assumed this was due to the more advanced medical technology and better medical conditions in the U.S., particularly in terms of early detection, diagnosis, and treatment. However, a deeper look into the specific data revealed some very interesting facts.

Particularly noteworthy are the cases of breast cancer and prostate cancer. These cancers show a significant difference in incidence rates between the two countries: in China, the incidence rate of breast cancer is 22.1 per 100,000, compared to 92.9 per 100,000 in the U.S.; prostate cancer has an incidence rate of 5.3 per 100,000 in China versus 98.2 per 100,000 in the U.S. Since the 5-year survival rates for these cancers are much higher than for other types, this discrepancy significantly widens the gap in the 5-year survival rates between the two countries.

Excluding these two cancers from the comparison, the 5-year survival rates for cancer in China and the U.S. are 25% and 33%, respectively, significantly narrowing the gap. Moreover, when comparing the mortality rates of these cancers, it is found that China's rates are notably lower than those in the U.S., with breast cancer mortality rates of 5.4 per 100,000 in China and 14.9 per 100,000 in the U.S.; prostate cancer mortality rates are 2.5 per 100,000 in China and 9.8 per 100,000 in the U.S. These results suggest that early detection, diagnosis, and treatment of breast and prostate cancer have not significantly improved outcomes.

B.   <u>Conducting prospective cohort studies to compare the incidence and mortality rates of cancer between screened and unscreened populations provides valuable insights.</u>

In the United States, a research study involved men aged 55 to 74 undergoing prostate cancer screening. The study included 38,340 men in the screening group who received annual PSA tests, and 38,345 men in the control group who did not undergo PSA testing. After a 10-year follow-up, 92% of participants completed the study, and 57% completed a 13-year follow-up. The results showed that the incidence of prostate cancer in the screening group was 108.4 cases per 100,000 person-years, compared to 97.1 cases per 100,000 person-years in the control group, an increase of 12%. However, the mortality rates from prostate cancer were

3.7 per 100,000 person-years in the screening group and 3.4 per 100,000 person-years in the control group, showing no significant difference between the two groups.

Another study, known as the ERSPC, was conducted across seven European countries involving 182,000 men aged 50 to 74, with 162,243 men aged between 59 and 69. In this study, 72,890 men underwent PSA screening every four years, while the rest did not. After a 9-year follow-up, the cumulative incidence of prostate cancer was 8.2% in the screening group and 4.8% in the non-screening group, a significant difference. However, the screening group saw a 20% reduction in the rate of death from prostate cancer compared to the control group. Despite this, the actual difference in mortality rates over the 9 years was only 0.071%, suggesting that the real-world impact of early diagnosis and treatment might be limited.

These studies provide important information about prostate cancer screening, especially valuable in assessing the necessity and effectiveness of screening. The findings indicate that while screening may increase the rate of diagnosed cases, its impact on reducing mortality is not significant, suggesting a need for cautious promotion of prostate cancer screening.

C.   <u>Examining non-cancer deceased individuals or general medical patients for cancerous lesions reveals significant findings.</u>

In pathological examinations of thyroid tissue from individuals who died from non-thyroid cancer causes, 36% were found to have cancerous lesions. This percentage increases when tissue sections are cut thinner, to 0.5mm. Furthermore, pathological examinations of breast tissue from deceased women aged 40 to 50 who did not die from cancer showed that 40% had breast cancer lesions. In Japan, prostate tissue examinations of 525 men who died accidentally revealed that 82% of those aged 70 and above had prostate cancer, with a detection rate of 46% among those aged 50 to 59, and even an 8% detection rate in men as young as 20.

These data suggest that with advancements in diagnostic technologies, more examinations are likely to detect more cases of cancer. For instance, lung CT scans in a smoking population aged 50 reveal pulmonary nodules in 50% of the cases, yet based on a 10-year mortality risk, 96.4% of these nodules are not fatal; similarly, in non-smokers, 15% are likely to show pulmonary nodules on CT scans, with 99.3% being non-fatal. Similar findings are reported with CT scans of the kidneys and liver. Ultrasound screenings of the thyroid in the same demographic reveal suspected cancerous lesions in two-thirds of individuals. Generally, these incidental findings, known as incidentalomas, indicate a less than 1% ten-year mortality rate for the 50-year-old demographic, excluding smokers.

Therefore, there are grounds to question the positive impact of early detection and treatment on the prognosis of cancer patients, especially in the context of prevalent overtreatment in cancer care. Early detection and treatment do not necessarily improve survival rates and may instead reduce quality of life due to the side effects of treatment.

1.6 Patients' Tendency to Not Participate in Decision-Making During Treatment

In the current medical system, many patients tend to remain passive during their treatment process, often relying entirely on their doctor's recommendations without asking questions. Due to time constraints or communication styles, doctors may not fully explain all treatment options, or may not present the information in a way that's easily understandable for patients. In some cultural contexts, patients might refrain from expressing their views or doubts out of high respect for medical professionals. Additionally, patients with limited education or health literacy may find it challenging to understand complex medical information, which can deter them from participating in decision-making. Economic status and insurance limitations can also influence treatment choices. Without support from family or other advocates, patients might not realize that they can or should have a say in their treatment decisions.

This phenomenon of patient non-participation is even more pronounced in the field of cancer treatment. Cancer treatment often involves complex medical procedures and multiple treatment options, making it particularly difficult for patients to understand and evaluate all available choices. Furthermore, the severity of cancer can induce fear and uncertainty, leading patients to rely more on the professional judgment of their doctors rather than actively engaging in decision-making.

Indeed, the lack of patient involvement in cancer treatment decisions can have long-term consequences. The problem of overtreatment in cancer is difficult to address, and the healthcare system does not seem to encourage active patient participation. Although doctors' concerns about over-intervention are understandable, even the NCCN guidelines recommend that patients communicate with their treatment teams and consider their advice. Additionally, in pharmaceutical development, patient perspectives are often overlooked, especially evident in the marketing of prescription drugs where pharmaceutical companies view doctors as their primary customers, despite the medications being intended for patients.

This book aims to change this status quo by encouraging and guiding cancer patients to actively participate in their treatment decisions. By providing necessary information and tools, this book helps patients gain a basic understanding of cancer treatments, comprehend the pros and cons of various options, and thus communicate more effectively with their doctors to make decisions that better suit their individual health conditions and long-term interests.

Patients should have the right and opportunity to understand all viable treatment options, including the potential risks and benefits of each. Active participation not only helps patients make choices that better meet their individual needs but also enhances overall satisfaction and effectiveness of the treatment. Therefore, having a voice in cancer treatment is not only a patient's right but also a critical factor in improving treatment outcomes.

2. FIRST PRINCIPLES AND REDUCTIONISM

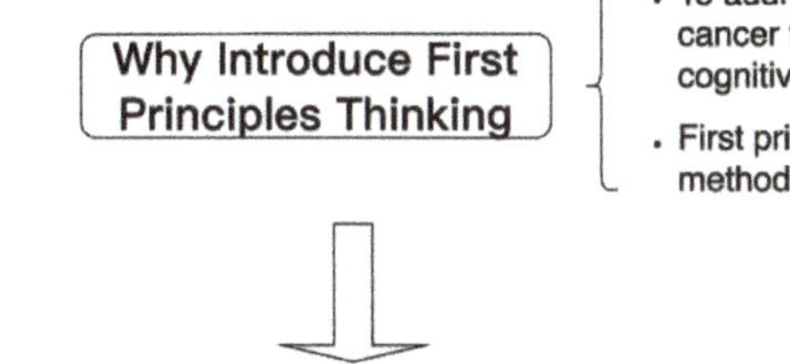

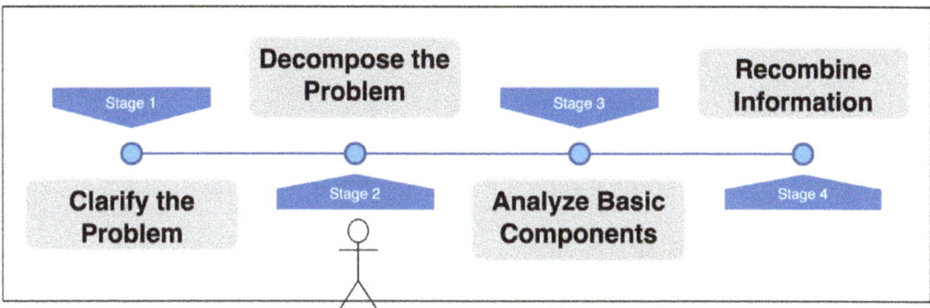

Adjustment in Applying First Principles to Cancer:
The medical community is caught in a reductionism trap with complex cancer issues.
It is necessary to focus the decomposition of the problem at the **cellular level** rather than the more complex molecular level.

Just as SpaceX has developed reusable rockets, the field of cancer treatment needs to break from tradition and find truly effective treatments. By applying first principles—starting from basic principles and reevaluating existing treatment methods—we might find more effective treatment options. This allows patients to precisely choose the most beneficial treatment from the standard options recommended by doctors. This is not just a choice of treatment but a respect for and responsibility towards life.

2.1 What Are First Principles?

First-principles thinking is a powerful method used to solve complex problems and unleash creativity. Often referred to as "reasoning from first principles," this approach involves breaking down complex issues into their most fundamental elements and then reconstructing them from scratch. It's a valuable way to foster independent thinking, tap into deep creative potential, and transition from linear to nonlinear innovation.

Historically adopted by thinkers like Aristotle and utilized by modern visionaries such as Elon Musk and Charlie Munger, this method allows them to see through flawed reasoning and inadequate analogies, discovering opportunities that others overlook.

Richard Feynman once remarked, "People don't learn by understanding; they learn in other ways—by rote or otherwise. Their knowledge is so fragile!" This statement underscores the importance of independent thinking.

The core concept is that a first principle is a basic assumption or proposition that exists independently and cannot be deduced from any other proposition or assumption. Aristotle discussed first principles by saying, "In every systematic inquiry where there are first principles, or causes, or elements, knowledge and science result from acquiring knowledge of these; for we think we know something only when we have grasped the primary causes, the primary principles, all the way to the elements." He later connected this concept with knowledge, defining a first principle as "the first basis from which a thing is known."

Pursuing first-principles thinking is not limited to philosophy; it's a common practice among great thinkers. Reasoning from first principles eliminates assumptions and traditions, leaving only the essential elements. This mode of thinking is crucial for enhancing cognitive abilities, as it helps identify where reasoning by analogy might lead to errors.

First Principles Thinking is a philosophical approach that involves breaking down complex problems into their most basic components. It involves exploring the 'first principles' or fundamental truths of a problem or situation, then rebuilding it from the ground up. This method encourages us to question assumptions, rethink norms, and explore new possibilities unrestricted by existing models or beliefs.

Elon Musk is renowned for his first-principles thinking, making him one of the most innovative entrepreneurs globally. Musk's success lies not just in his innovative ideas but in his way of thinking:

"People often process thoughts constrained by tradition or past experiences. They seldom try to view problems from the perspective of first principles. They might say, 'We do it this way because it's always been done this way.' Or they might avoid trying something new because 'no one has ever done it, so it must not be possible.' This way of thinking is flawed. It's crucial to build your reasoning from the ground up—as they say in physics, 'from first principles.' You need to examine the basic facts and build your reasoning from these facts to see if your conclusions align with past practices."

Musk's method starts with known truths rather than relying on intuition. The challenge with this approach is that our knowledge is limited, making intuition unreliable. When tackling complex problems like building rockets, he always starts from the first principles. Larry Page described Musk's thought process as follows: "What are the underlying physical principles? What are the time and cost involved? How can costs be reduced? This requires a certain degree of engineering and physical knowledge to make informed decisions. Elon has this understanding, as well as expertise in business, organization, and leadership."

Rockets are notoriously expensive, which posed a barrier to Musk's exploration of Mars. To address this, Musk asked the key question: "What materials make up a rocket? Aerospace-grade aluminum alloys, titanium, copper, and carbon fiber. What is the market value of these materials?" He was surprised to find that the material cost of a rocket was only about two percent of its typical sale price.

So, why is space travel so expensive? Musk, a self-taught polymath with degrees in economics and physics, delved into rocket science. He realized that the high cost of launching rockets stemmed from a way of thinking incompatible with first principles. This insight led him to found SpaceX and start building rockets from scratch.

In an interview with Kevin Rose, Musk emphasized the importance of reasoning from first principles rather than relying on analogies: "Reasoning from first principles rather than by analogy is crucial. Our typical approach is to reason by analogy, comparing existing experiences or practices with past situations. This method is easier than reasoning from first principles, which requires breaking down concepts into fundamental truths and then building from there. It demands more mental effort."

Musk demonstrated how SpaceX applies first principles to drive innovation at a lower cost: "Some might think battery packs are inherently expensive and will remain so due to historical trends. However, this is a mistaken assumption. If we approach every new idea this way, progress will be hindered. You can't dismiss new inventions by saying 'no one wants cars because horses are good enough.' By breaking down the components and costs of battery packs into their material constituents, we can discover innovative ways to manufacture batteries much cheaper than expected."

2.2 The Process of First Principles Thinking and Its Distinction from Reductionism

First principles thinking is a powerful method for solving problems. In real life, whether it's completing a task or solving a problem, there are often unsatisfactory aspects, especially when dealing with complex issues. Traditional solutions have not brought significant improvements over time, making first principles thinking particularly important. It challenges conventional habits and viewpoints, breaks down problems, and starts from the most basic elements, using fundamental laws to construct a complete analytical model. This deductive logic process ensures the correctness and completeness of the analytical model. Ultimately, this new model helps us find the real answers to problems.

At its core, thinking from first principles seems very intuitive. However, while this principle appears simple, it is quite challenging to implement in practice.

The importance of first principles thinking in analysis lies not only in its ability to help us break down data but also in encouraging us to question and understand the fundamental elements that constitute the data. This method includes the following key steps:

1) **Clarify the Problem:** All analysis should start with a clear definition of the problem. Before beginning the analysis, it is essential to clearly define the problem or concept. This provides a clear direction for subsequent steps and ensures the focus of the work is correct. Sometimes it's challenging to identify the real problem, as this requires going beyond what we consider "obvious."

2) **Decompose the Problem:** Once the real problem to be solved is identified, the next step is to break it down. What components make up the problem or idea? How are these parts connected? This step may involve research, interviews, and a deep understanding of the

problem. This process can take a long time and may require multiple iterations, so patience is necessary. This step is like dissecting a complex machine into its basic parts.

3) **Analyze Basic Components:** After breaking down the problem, the next step is to understand these basic elements and how they interact. At this stage, distinguishing between assumptions and fundamental truths becomes very important. Each component should be carefully examined, questioned, and understood. You need to constantly question all assumptions, asking yourself, "Is this true?" or "Is this just my assumption?" During this stage, analysts challenge existing assumptions and models, asking fundamental "why" and "how" questions to reveal the real drivers behind observed trends and patterns.

4) **Recombine Information:** After completing this extensive task, you should have a clear understanding of the basic elements and their interrelationships. The final step is to synthesize this information. Here, the problem or idea is reconstructed from a new perspective, and you start looking for the right solutions to address these components and issues. Because only with a deep understanding of the basic facts can these become the building blocks for new solutions, new business models, or insights. In this recombination phase, true innovation thrives because people are no longer bound by traditional models or assumptions but focus on the pure problem rather than the assumptions.

In summary, starting from scratch and using insights gained from basic elements and questioning assumptions, analysts can build a more accurate and nuanced analytical model.

First principles thinking is indeed a powerful method that helps us fundamentally understand and solve problems. Unlike relying on traditional analogies, precedents, corrective methods, or conventional wisdom, this approach encourages us to directly explore the essence of a problem—the "real issue"—and analyze it without bias or preconceived notions. By breaking down the problem into its basic elements, we can adopt a fresh perspective, start from scratch, and innovate one element at a time.

In the second phase, breaking down the problem, it's quite easy to make mistakes. Theoretically, matter can be infinitely decomposed, even down to the atomic level, and with technological advances, it might be possible to break it down even further. At this stage, it's easy to fall into a reductionist mindset. For example, in the case of SpaceX, first principles analysis determined that the basic components of rockets are the rocket parts themselves, without needing to analyze the molecular structure of the fuel or the molecular level of materials.

Reductionism is a deeply ingrained way of thinking, fundamentally about breaking down a whole object into smaller parts. As technology advances, humans can explore finer levels, thus introducing reductionism to complex levels. However, this approach has a significant problem: it tends to overlook complexity. In physics, it's easy to see the whole as composed of parts, but in complex fields like medicine, the parts often exceed the sum of the whole.

In physics, systems are often seen as the simple sum of their parts, meaning the properties and functions of the whole can be directly derived from its components. This viewpoint reflects the reductionism in physics, which involves understanding the entire system by studying its basic building units.

However, in medicine and other complex scientific fields, the situation is usually more complicated. The systems studied in these fields, such as organisms, ecosystems, or social systems, exhibit high degrees of non-linearity and interaction, making the properties of the whole more than just a simple sum of its parts. This phenomenon, known as "the whole is greater than the sum of its parts," means that the behavior and characteristics of the whole cannot be fully predicted by analyzing its components.

For example, in an organism, the behavior of a single cell or molecule may have entirely different effects within the entire organism because they interact within a complex biological feedback and regulatory network. Therefore, simply understanding the functions of parts, like cells or organs, cannot fully explain or treat diseases involving the entire biological system.

Modern medicine often finds itself entrenched in a reductionist approach, focusing intensely on the minutest details. To navigate away from this, employing first principles is essential. Both first principles and reductionism involve breaking concepts down to their fundamental elements. However, the crucial difference lies in their scope and application. First principles focus on basic elements at a level manageable and predictable by the thinker, whereas reductionism delves into the most minute details observable by humans.

In the fourth phase, the critical stage of innovation, in a whole problem composed of basic parts, the true rule is unique or self-evident. This rule (including causality) is the first principle. Like physical laws, this rule can often be described using mathematical models, allowing analysts using first principles to construct a more accurate and nuanced analytical model.

Overall, although first principles and reductionism do not differ in the pursuit of finer levels, first principles are more effective in solving complex problems. Its way of thinking is correct in terms of causality and significantly different from traditional solutions.

To illustrate the steps of first principles thinking, a simple flowchart can be designed. Here's a basic example:

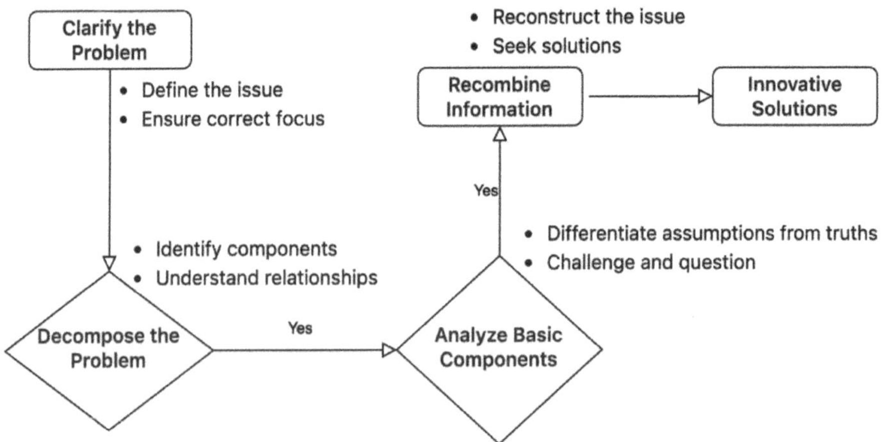

3. HOW TO ANALYZE CANCER TREATMENT USING FIRST PRINCIPLES

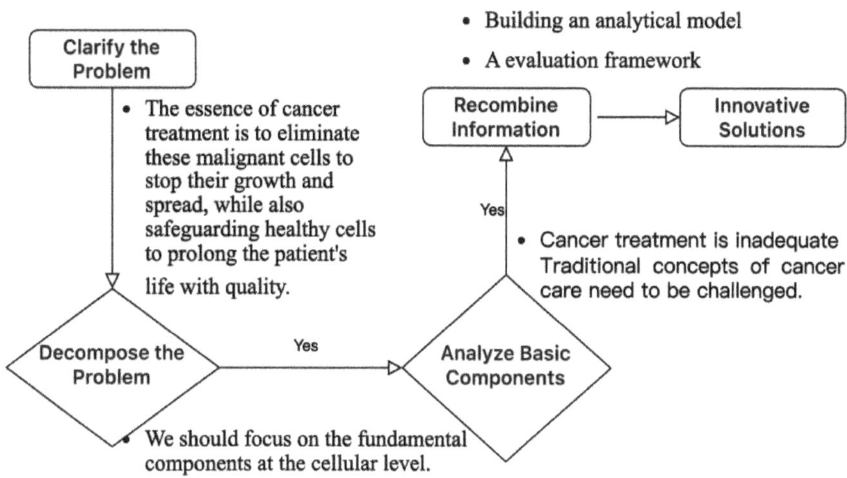

In discussing cancer, our precise understanding is at the cellular level rather than the more microscopic molecular level. Contrarily, modern medicine's pursuit of complex fields like molecular biology or genetics often demands in-depth research. Unless a certain level of complexity is achieved, such studies may not gain peer recognition, even though they could significantly aid in addressing real-world medical issues.

The current landscape of cancer treatment and research faces the challenge of overly pursuing technical complexity at the expense of practicality. By reexamining the causes and progression of cancer through the lens of first principles, we can develop more concrete treatment strategies at the cellular level.

Analyzing cancer treatment using first principles allows us to break down the problem into basic facts and principles, and then build reasoning and solutions based on these foundations. This approach helps us break free from traditional thought patterns and experiential limitations, finding more innovative and effective treatment methods.

Of course, due to strict regulations in the medical field, innovative treatment methods not approved by regulatory bodies cannot be applied clinically. Cancer patients themselves also struggle to push for the approval of new treatments. However, we can still use first principles to select suitable and approved therapies that meet our treatment goals.

3.1 Identifying the Real Problem

Cancer is a disease marked by the uncontrolled growth and spread of malignant cells that invade and gradually destroy healthy tissues and organs, potentially leading to death. Thus, the essence of cancer treatment is to eliminate these malignant cells to stop their growth and spread, while also safeguarding healthy cells to prolong the patient's life with quality.

In the medical field, there is a viewpoint that truly curing cancer requires a deep understanding of its causes and main contributing factors. Proponents believe that understanding the origins of the disease not only helps in evaluating existing treatments but could also guide the development of more effective strategies.

However, when determining how to tackle cancer, we do not necessarily need a complete understanding of all the reasons behind its occurrence and its main triggers. Similar to car repairs, knowing the cause of a malfunction may not directly aid the repair process, as the methods are often straightforward and uniform, typically involving the replacement of damaged parts. The same logic applies to cancer treatment; our primary focus should not be on exploring why cells lose control over growth but rather on how to eliminate malignant cells to prevent their growth and spread, while protecting healthy cells to extend the patient's life with quality. This approach is more direct and practical, potentially better suited for addressing the urgent and complex medical challenge of cancer.

3.2 Breaking Down the Real Problem

Identifying the real issue in cancer treatment is straightforward: we need the most effective methods to eliminate cancer cells while protecting healthy ones, ultimately extending the patient's quality of life. However, a deeper analysis of this issue requires a more comprehensive approach. We can start with the following basic elements:

Nature of Cancer: Cancer is a disease caused by abnormal cell growth, often rooted in mutations and uncontrolled growth of cellular genetic material.

Treatment Goals: The primary goal is to eliminate or inhibit the growth of abnormal cells to prevent the spread and recurrence of cancer, thereby extending the patient's quality of life.

Treatment Methods: Current methods include chemotherapy, radiation, surgery, and targeted therapy. Different strategies are employed depending on the type and stage of cancer.

We can break down the problem of cancer treatment into more specific questions:

1) How can we accurately identify and locate cancer cells for targeted treatment?
2) Can we develop new treatment methods that intervene based on specific characteristics of cancer cells?
3) How can we maximize treatment effectiveness while minimizing side effects and the risk of damaging healthy cells?

4)   The ultimate goal of cancer treatment is to extend the patient's quality of life, not just to eliminate cancer cells. Are current treatment methods aligned with this goal?

Clearly, these questions center on how to effectively eliminate cancer cells and extend the patient's life with quality.

Numerous issues exist in current cancer treatments, both in the development of new therapies and in the clinical application of approved treatments. Firstly, most cancer therapies listed in treatment guidelines focus on the patient's short-term benefits. Secondly, the majority of cancer treatments, especially drug therapies, are related to genetic mutations and targets. Their effects are primarily at the molecular level below the cell, and they do not linearly correlate with effective cancer cell elimination, rendering them ineffective in many cases. Thirdly, new cancer therapies focus on complex and cutting-edge technologies, pushing simple and practical treatments out of the options for cancer care. Fourthly, guided by these guidelines, doctors tend to overtreat patients.

The root of these issues lies in the medical community's (including both researchers developing therapies and doctors administering treatments) misplacement of the basic components of cancer treatment, attempting to treat cancer by manipulating molecular-level variables. However, molecular-level therapies have led to many unpredictable phenomena. Breaking down the problem of cancer treatment to the cellular level is appropriate, but positioning the basic components at the genetic or even molecular level introduces complexities far greater than the problems it solves. The transmission of effects from genes to cells is not linear, and currently, humans cannot effectively regulate cell behavior by adjusting genes. Therefore, in addressing cancer treatment, we should focus on the fundamental components at the cellular level, including cancer cells, normal cells, and the immune system.

3.3 Analyzing the Fundamental Components

At this stage, we begin by posing the following questions:

1) What is the current level of cancer treatment? In reality, it is not very high.

2) Does relying on current medical research help develop better cancer treatment plans? In fact, this task is extremely challenging because reductionist thinking still prevails in the medical community.

3) In the existing healthcare system, do doctors always adopt the best interest of the patients? Not necessarily, it is largely a random process, and overtreatment is a significant issue.

4) In the existing treatment options, can cancer patients choose the plan that maximizes their long-term benefits? Due to a general lack of necessary scientific knowledge, patients are easily influenced by the healthcare system, and most mistakenly believe that the doctor's decision is optimal.

In the section on the current state of cancer treatment, we have identified two basic facts: First, the level of cancer treatment does not vary significantly between countries, and the outcomes in developed countries with advanced medical technology are not superior to those in developing countries. Second, the existing medical system tends to overtreat and does not prioritize the long-term interests of cancer patients.

The root cause of these facts is that the existing medical system does not address the real issues we identified earlier, or that the current cancer treatments are not the best solutions to the cancer problem.

From several typical first principles cases, we know that traditional solutions have not brought significant improvements over a long period. This is where the first principles become particularly important. They challenge conventional habits and views, break down problems, and start with the most basic elements, using fundamental laws to build a comprehensive analytical model. This is a deductive logic process that ensures the correctness and completeness of the analytical model. Ultimately, through this new analytical model, we can find the real answers to the problems. We find that existing cancer treatments have not brought significant improvements; therefore, we need to use the laws of disease to construct a comprehensive analytical model above the cellular level. Current technology allows humans to directly manipulate cells and accurately predict outcomes. By focusing on the cellular level as the fundamental component of cancer issues, we establish a solid foundation for the next steps. This approach is logically sound and reduces as much uncertainty as possible in the cancer treatment process.

3.4 Reassembling Information

At the cellular level, the characteristics of cancer cells include uncontrolled growth. For solid tumors, cancer cells cluster together, generate their own blood vessels to supply nutrients, and usurp the physical space of normal cells while evading the immune system's surveillance. There are many methods to eliminate cancer cells, but the most effective treatment is often the simplest. It is also necessary to consider the side effects of the treatment. With this information, we can be selective, choosing the existing cancer treatment method that most efficiently addresses our problems. Furthermore, we are not limited to one method; we might choose multiple therapies and combine them into a comprehensive treatment plan.

As a cancer patient reading this section of the book, you might use first principles to analyze the treatment plan your doctor has given you, or to explore other treatment options your doctor hasn't mentioned. However, applying first principles is not so straightforward; it requires more information for validation and understanding, enabling even those without extensive medical knowledge to navigate their cancer treatment journey using first principles.

Building an analytical model based on first principles is crucial. It uses self-evident laws and the most basic components to construct a framework for cancer treatment. In this book, I propose a life model that links cancer and aging, where part of the analysis will use the logical completeness of mathematics to address issues like treatment principles and resistance in cancer. This approach simplifies the complex problem of cancer treatment.

I believe that through mathematical models, we can construct a comprehensive framework for evaluating cancer treatments. While first principles themselves are a way of thinking and do not directly lead to advances in cancer treatment technology, we can use the comprehensive evaluation framework built on first principles to guide patients in choosing the best treatment options that are truly beneficial for them. Researchers can also use this framework to develop innovative cancer treatments.

PART TWO: THE ESSENCE OF CANCER TREATMENT (CANCER AND AGING IN THE LIFE MODEL)

"Living organisms avoid the decline into thermodynamic equilibrium by maintaining negative entropy through homeostasis in an open system."

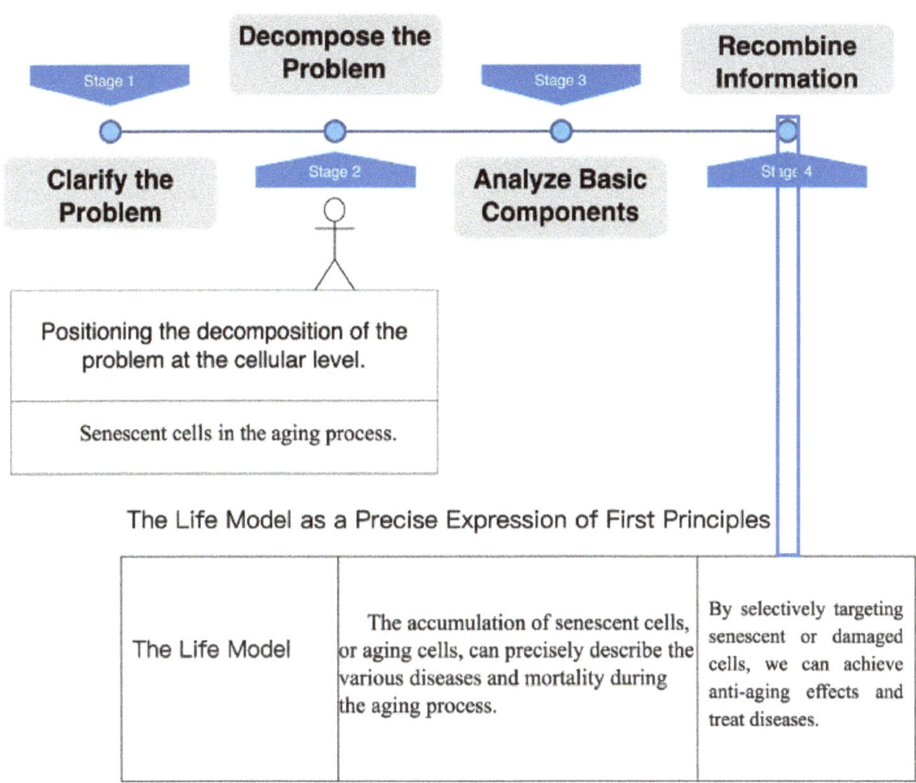

The Life Model as a Precise Expression of First Principles

The Life Model	The accumulation of senescent cells, or aging cells, can precisely describe the various diseases and mortality during the aging process.	By selectively targeting senescent or damaged cells, we can achieve anti-aging effects and treat diseases.

In the previous chapter, we analyzed the issues of cancer treatment using first principles, particularly focusing on the second step where we positioned the fundamental components at the cellular level. This step is crucial for introducing first principles into solving cancer treatment problems because it allows us to progress to the fourth step. Here, we start from these basic components to construct a new analytical model. This step requires that the basic components be at a level where humans can manipulate them and anticipate the outcomes. Positioning the basic components at the cellular level also serves as a way to correct the overly reductionist trend in medical research.

The fourth step of first principles involves building a new analytical model from the basic components and deriving new insights. One of the most convenient methods to complete this process is by establishing mathematical models. Mathematical models have at least three advantages when describing complex biological processes: first, their assumptions are clearly articulated in mathematical language; second, their logical reasoning is rigorous and precise, helping prevent flaws and fallacies; third, existing mathematical models or theorems can be applied to deduce new results, achieving conclusions that are difficult or impossible to reach through intuition alone. It can be said that mathematical models in biology represent the most precise expression of first principles in the field.

4.1 Constructing a Life model

According to Erwin Schrödinger, life counteracts the increase in entropy prescribed by the second law of thermodynamics by absorbing energy to maintain or reduce its entropy, a concept he termed negative entropy. However, this idea of negative entropy broadly outlines rather than concretely defines the entire process of life. If we consider an organism as entirely made up of cells, entropy then measures the level of orderliness within the organism. An increase in entropy indicates a shift from order to disorder, thus the overall orderliness of cells mirrors the organism's state of order. When dysfunctional cells such as senescent or cancerous cells appear, they disrupt this order, reducing the organism's orderliness. Let's categorize these inefficient or disorder-causing cells as aging cells, which include all types of dysfunctional and malignantly proliferating cells, primarily affecting the organism through spatial occupation and disruption of order. The ratio of aging cells to the total number of cells serves as an intuitive measure of the increase in entropy within the organism.

We can then formulate a life model[1]: the human body consists of approximately 50 trillion (50×10^{12}) cells. When the proportion of dysfunctional aging cells, such as senescent cells, reaches a certain threshold, the individual's systemic functions deteriorate, leading to death. In this model, a localized excess of dysfunctional cells beyond a certain limit signals the onset of disease. The body's natural mechanisms, particularly the immune system, strive to slow down or minimize the accumulation of these aging cells.

---

[1] In the Further Readingsection of this book, we provide a detailed process for building mathematical models of life, aimed at readers with a mathematical background.

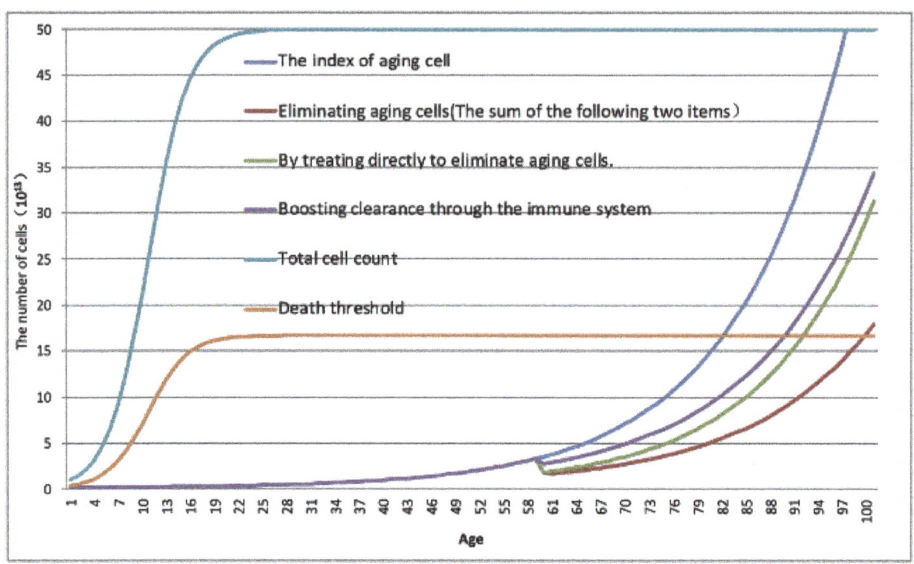

The selective removal of aging cells can consistently lower the aging cell index, which is calculated as the ratio of aging cells to the total cell count. This elimination process includes direct removal via medical interventions and clearance through enhanced immune functions. In this context, aging cells, or senescent cells, encompass both dysfunctional cells and cancer cells.

From birth, our body's cells are subjected to various damages due to environmental or systemic factors. Once these damages reach a certain threshold, cells age and are targeted for clearance by the immune system. However, this clearance process is not entirely efficient. We use the immune system's ability to eliminate cancer cells as a model to understand its capacity to clear aging cells. This capacity diminishes over time, as suggested by the immunoediting hypothesis, which proposes that cancer cells eventually evade the immune system because its clearance ability weakens with age. This variable is crucial as it reflects the impact of aging on the immune system and the potential long-term effects of artificially enhancing the immune system on the body's ability to eliminate aging cells.

Cells in the body do not become senescent at a predetermined time but accumulate damage over time, leading to senescence. This damage likely affects all cells, not just a specific subset. As time passes, the number of senescent cells increases, accelerating the aging process.

In the animal kingdom, a noticeable pattern emerges: the larger an adult animal is, the longer its maximum lifespan tends to be. The size of an adult animal can explain about 63% of its maximum lifespan variability. Assuming that an animal dies when a certain proportion of its cells become senescent, and considering that all animals share the same rate of cellular damage, immune capacity, and rate of immune function decline, an animal's lifespan would primarily depend on its size.

This model effectively explains why larger animals tend to live longer: they have more total cells as adults, requiring a greater number of senescent cells to reach a critical level that leads to death. Since the accumulation of senescent cells is solely time-dependent and not cleared efficiently, larger animals take longer to reach the critical proportion of senescent cells, thereby extending their lifespan.

4.2 Treatment or Prevention of Diseases

According to physical laws, when an animal falls ill, it indicates that some of its cells are no longer functioning correctly. The strategy to treat diseases typically involves either repairing these dysfunctional cells or removing and replacing them with new ones. In humans, for instance, when diseases occur—such as cells becoming inactive or deteriorating—these cells are considered senescent in our model. So, how do we address these diseases? According to physical laws, we can only remove these damaged cells, since repairing them is nearly impossible for humans. We then rely on the body's natural mechanisms, particularly using remaining stem cells, to regenerate healthy cells to replace the ones that have been removed. Our model simplifies this by assuming that stem cell regeneration automatically occurs after the damaged cells are cleared. Since stem cells regenerate younger and healthier cells, if this regeneration can occur naturally without other limitations, then, according to our model, once the senescent cells are cleared, everything else follows naturally.

Let's consider chronic diseases like diabetes, cancer, or Alzheimer's disease, where a patient's accumulation of senescent cells grows exponentially. Without intervention, the patient is likely to have a shorter lifespan compared to a healthy individual. If we apply effective treatment, this is reflected in the backward shift of the age-related cell accumulation curve.

According to our model, there are two main types of treatments: 1) directly clearing senescent cells, and 2) enhancing immune capacity, which improves the clearance of senescent cells. Either approach effectively shifts the senescent cell accumulation curve backward, thus delaying the intersection with the death threshold and extending the patient's lifespan. Many treatments can achieve both—directly clearing senescent cells and boosting immune capacity. For example, removing senescent cells might expose antigens to the immune system, thereby enhancing its capacity to clear more senescent cells, pushing the curve even further back and extending lifespan even more.

In practice, tumor ablation can increase patient survival; similarly, clearing senescent cells has been shown to extend the lifespan in animals. These real-world examples support our model's predictions.

4.3 The Life Model as a Precise Expression of First Principles

My life model is categorized under systems biology, a branch of complex science that views biological entities as complex adaptive systems. Contemporary medical research often adopts a reductionist approach, focusing on the most fundamental components—molecules—to understand life processes and disease states. This method has led to significant discoveries about molecular mechanisms and new drug targets. However, it has critical shortcomings:

1) **Neglecting Complexity:** Biological systems are intricate and dynamic. A change in a single molecule may not sufficiently explain alterations in the entire system. Diseases typically arise from the interplay of multiple factors, which reductionism may fail to capture, overlooking the complexity at the system level.

2) **Overlooking Environmental Factors:** Disease onset is influenced not only by molecular and genetic factors but also by environmental,

lifestyle, and psychological factors. An excessive focus on the molecular level can lead to the neglect of these crucial external influences.

3) **Limitations of Disease Models:** Molecular-level disease studies often rely on simplified models like cell cultures or animal models, which may not fully capture the complexity of human diseases, thus limiting the relevance of research findings.

4) **Individual Differences in Treatment:** People may respond differently to **treatments** even if they target the same molecular pathways. Reductionism struggles to account for these individual variations.

While molecular research has propelled forward our understanding and treatment of diseases, there is a growing shift towards a systems biology approach. This method integrates data across various biological levels—from molecules to the whole organism—and considers genetic, environmental, and lifestyle factors, aiming for a comprehensive understanding of diseases. Nevertheless, current systems biology still tends to follow a reductionist trajectory, trying to exhaustively map all variable relationships, which seems impractical.

Aiming for a simpler, more elegant theory, akin to Schrödinger's concept of negative entropy, might be more appropriate for systems biology than attempting to construct a highly complex model.

Upon reviewing the drug development process, it's clear that most new drugs stem from detailed molecular studies, which seems to validate reductionism. However, when assessing the effectiveness of current medical treatments, the small number of curable diseases compared to the vast array of human diseases suggests that new research approaches are necessary.

Similar to how mathematical modeling in complex sciences often simplifies systems to emphasize key variables, systems biology should also focus on levels where human intervention can be most effective. If research at one level becomes too complex, we should consider moving to a more manageable level. For instance, if genomic research proves too intricate, shifting focus to the proteomic or even cellular level might be beneficial. At the cellular level, we can focus on the average effects of genes and proteins rather than on specific variables.

In the application of first principles, the second step is crucial: breaking down the problem into its fundamental components. In disease research, applying first principles correctly requires a clear identification of these basic components, which should be controllable by humans and yield predictable outcomes. Choosing the cellular level as the fundamental component in your life model is an apt application of these principles.

Utilizing mathematical models to describe the complex processes of biology offers several advantages. Firstly, the assumptions made are articulated clearly in mathematical language, which helps ensure that the analysis starts from a clear and consistent base. Secondly, the reasoning is tight and precise, effectively preventing errors and fallacies, thus ensuring the accuracy of the deductions. Lastly, existing mathematical models or theorems can be used to derive new results, reaching conclusions that might be difficult or impossible to obtain through intuition alone.

Therefore, the life model is not just a theoretical framework; it is a precise and practical expression of first principles in biology. This approach helps us gain a deeper understanding of the essence of diseases like cancer and provides a more scientific and precise foundation for treatment.

5. CANCER AS A PART OF AGING

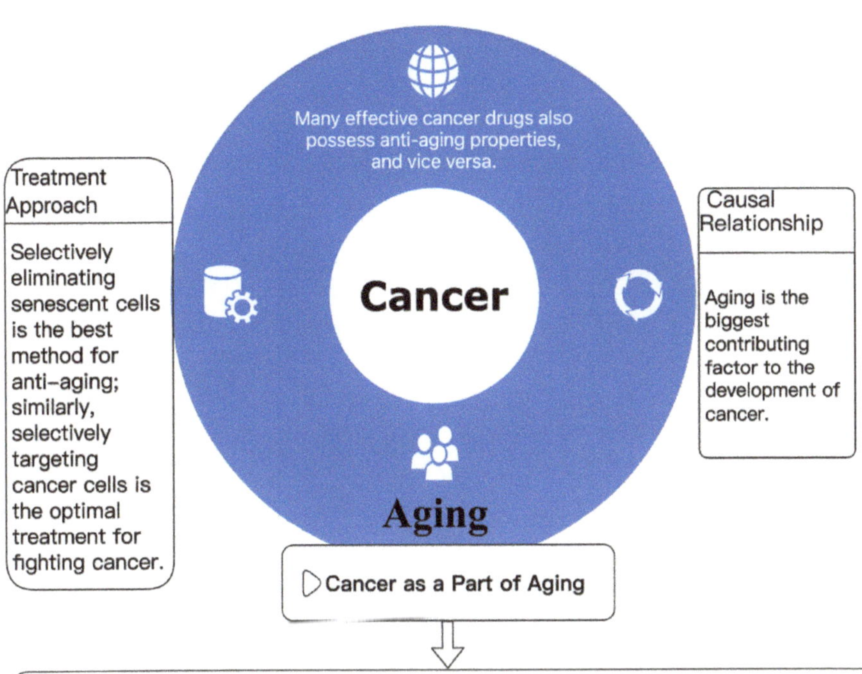

	Insights from Anti-Aging Strategies for Cancer Treatment
1	Clearing cancer cells effectively is crucial; however, aiming for 100% clearance is unrealistic and can lead to overtreatment.
2	Viewing cancer as a manageable chronic condition, similar to aging, suggests that continuous treatment could be more effective than attempting complete eradication at once.
3	The primary goal of cancer treatment should be to maintain long-term, high-quality life, rather than focusing solely on immediate eradication or preventing recurrence.
4	Cancer treatments should prioritize minimizing side effects to preserve overall long-term quality of life, similar to criteria used in anti-aging therapies.
5	Drugs effective in anti-aging may also offer anti-cancer benefits, suggesting that treatments aligning with both goals could be more beneficial and appropriate.

5.1 The Connection Between Cancer and Aging

Data on cancer indicates a direct correlation with aging. In countries with aging populations, cancer incidence is significantly higher than in younger populations. While age-adjusted incidence rates vary significantly between countries, possibly due to early detection, age-adjusted cancer mortality rates are relatively uniform worldwide, with most countries reporting 80 to 100 deaths per 100,000 people. This suggests that cancer is primarily related to aging.

If we consider cancer and aging as two types of diseases, we see many similarities between them, showing a strong equivalence. Researchers have identified common features such as genomic instability, epigenetic alterations, chronic inflammation, and dysbiosis as hallmarks of both aging and cancer. Some hallmarks of aging, such as loss of proteostasis, mitochondrial dysfunction, and altered intercellular communication, do not have direct counterparts in cancer markers but may contribute to specific cancer characteristics, thereby facilitating resistance to cell death, glycolytic metabolism, and tissue structure disruption.

Other aging hallmarks, like telomere attrition and stem cell exhaustion, clearly inhibit specific aspects of tumor development, such as replicative immortality and phenotypic plasticity. These are considered antagonistic hallmarks because they may represent instances of antagonistic pleiotropy. Dysfunctional autophagy and cellular senescence, two other hallmarks of aging, have context-dependent tumor-suppressive and tumor-promoting roles and thus warrant separate discussion.

Additionally, the equivalence or antagonism between aging-related nutrient sensing dysregulation and cancer-related metabolic disturbances is complex, necessitating research into the shared metabolic features of aging and cancer.

The failure of cancer immunosurveillance may be influenced by several aging characteristics. If this book compares cancer and aging, it might seem irrelevant to someone with cancer. However, understanding every relationship between aging and cancer could be crucial for someone who has cancer.

We need to carefully consider whether aging is a disease. Clearly, it is not; it is a natural law that everyone will experience. From the perspective of first principles, aging is a fundamental law that cannot and need not be broken down; it is not a problem but an axiom. On the other hand, cancer is a disease. Everyone ages, but not everyone develops cancer.

Human aging manifests uniformly: cellular senescence, tissue deformation, and organ dysfunction. Cancer also involves abnormal cell proliferation, tissue deformation, and organ dysfunction. Since aging encompasses more than cancer, we should not view them as two distinct diseases; rather, aging includes cancer, or cancer is a part of aging.

Given the current limitations of cancer treatments, which prevent cancer from becoming a chronic, manageable condition like an aging-related disease, if we view cancer as a part of aging, there should be therapies or drugs that can treat both cancer and counteract aging. Indeed, such a drug exists: metformin. Extensive clinical data has proven that metformin has low side effects and possesses both anticancer and anti-aging properties.

5.2 Cancer and Aging in the Life model

In our life model, aging is seen as the natural accumulation of senescent cells. When a certain proportion of these cells accumulates, it leads to the end of an individual's life. Some organs may have a higher proportion of these aged cells, indicating they have aged more significantly. Senescent cells are defined by their abnormal structure, diminished function, and their long-term occupation of space that could otherwise be occupied by new, healthy cells.

If we extend this definition to include cells that not only have an abnormal structure and completely lost function but also occupy space long-term without making way for new, healthy cells, and progressively destroy the surrounding tissue structure through proliferation, we describe the characteristics of cancer cells. Although cancer cells and senescent cells are not entirely the same, in our life model, they are indistinguishable to some extent. This means our life model can describe both the aging process and the cancer process.

In the Further Readingsection of this book, readers with a mathematical background will find that our life model primarily describes the quantity of senescent cells, including typical chronic disease-damaged cells and cancer cells. This implies that treatment variables in our life model mainly involve the clearance of senescent cells. We know that merely clearing damaged cells does not complete the treatment process, as the cleared cells leave behind physical space. Fortunately, organisms have an innate regenerative ability; once some cells are cleared, the organism automatically regenerates healthy cells to fill these spaces, a process that occurs without human intervention. Therefore, our life model is comprehensive, whether addressing aging or cancer.

For aging, the theoretical approach to anti-aging involves selectively clearing senescent cells. Effective methods include new therapies that directly clear these cells, reducing their proportion, or by stimulating the immune system to recognize and clear them. Selective clearance of senescent cells has become a hot topic in medical research and has shown promising results in animal studies.

For cancer, the treatment approach also involves selectively clearing cancer cells. Methods for clearing cancer cells include direct removal through surgery or ablation, or by stimulating the immune system to recognize and clear them. Nearly all cancer therapies currently employ one or a combination of these approaches.

Thus, our life model is fundamentally correct in describing both aging and cancer.

Considering metformin, which can both fight cancer and counteract aging, its ability to achieve these effects with minimal side effects primarily lies in its capacity to utilize the body's ROS to clear both senescent and cancer cells. Research indicates that metformin's benefits extend beyond traditional treatments, including weight loss, cancer prevention, anti-aging, anti-inflammatory effects, and even antiviral responses. While there is some controversy, some reports suggest that metformin may increase ROS levels, which could potentially trigger systemic anti-tumor immune responses and promote tissue regeneration. This hypothesis suggests that metformin's mechanism in treating various diseases might involve using ROS to clear damaged cells, contributing to its anti-aging and anti-cancer effects.

5.3 Insights from Anti-Aging Strategies for Cancer Treatment

Compared to cancer treatment, anti-aging is not as urgent, and because it involves longer clinical trials, there are not as many new therapies for anti-aging as there are for cancer treatment. Anti-aging focuses on the long term and rarely encounters common issues in cancer treatment such as treatment choice dilemmas and overtreatment. Given this, the few anti-aging approaches that align with first principles may offer insights for cancer treatment.

Currently, the focus in anti-aging is on a type of drug known as senolytics. These drugs can selectively clear senescent cells and have shown promising anti-aging effects in animal studies, with apparently low long-term side effects. Clearing senescent cells has gradually become a main focus in the development of anti-aging drugs.

Observing the development of senolytics as anti-aging agents offers several lessons for cancer treatment:

1) Effectively clearing cancer cells is key to fighting cancer, but aiming for 100% clearance is not necessary. As technology advances, our ability to identify and clear cancer cells will improve. However, since aging is inevitable, it is unlikely that all senescent cells can be cleared in the pursuit of anti-aging. In contrast, current cancer treatments often aim for 100% clearance of cancer cells, which is technically unfeasible and can lead to overtreatment.

2) Transforming cancer into a chronic condition, similar to anti-aging, suggests that cancer treatment should also be continuous. Just as we accept that senescent cells cannot be completely cleared at once and will accumulate over time, anti-aging measures are used continuously. In cancer treatment, both doctors and patients often aim for a one-time clearance of cancer cells, hoping they never return, which mirrors the first point. Our life model assumes that if the accumulation of senescent cells (or cancer cells) is kept at a low level, the organism can still survive, much like aging. Living with cancer is a more achievable treatment goal in reality.

3) The goal of treatment should be long-term high-quality life. Anti-aging aims to enable people to continue living high-quality lives. However, the goals of cancer treatment are often short-term. In choosing treatment methods, doctors might first aim to clear cancer cells completely; second, try to prevent recurrence, which severely opposes the concept of living with cancer; and third, completely disregard the patient's quality of life post-treatment. If the goal of cancer treatment is set on long-term high-quality life, most overtreatment can be avoided. Patients who read this book should aim

for a long-term high-quality life as their goal for cancer treatment, using first principles to choose appropriate treatment methods and influence doctors' decisions, which I believe can maximize treatment effectiveness.

4) More attention needs to be paid to side effects in cancer treatment decisions. Since anti-aging targets long-term high-quality life, any promising anti-aging therapy must be closely scrutinized for side effects, even minor ones, which could lead to the therapy being rejected. This is why the anti-aging industry is filled with a multitude of supplements that are explicitly free of side effects. In contrast, many cancer treatments involve toxic drugs and various cell-damaging therapies. While these are necessary to clear cancer cells, the side effects, which can harm the whole body or immune system, are often overlooked, resulting in treatments that sacrifice long-term quality of life for immediate effects.

5) Drugs that can counteract aging are likely to have anti-cancer effects. Conversely, if a cancer treatment does not have anti-aging effects, it should be carefully considered by patients, as it might be an inappropriate method. Although senolytics, drugs that selectively clear senescent cells, are not yet approved, many researchers have incorporated them into the development of anti-cancer drugs, indicating a general consensus that anti-aging drugs are likely to be effective against cancer. In the development of new cancer drugs, regardless of the inefficiency of traditional cancer drug development and the fact that existing cancer drugs may not provide long-term benefits, you do not need to wait for better, first-principle-aligned

cancer treatments. You can use metformin for cancer treatment, as extensive clinical data shows it can both counteract aging and fight cancer.

I recommend considering metformin for several compelling reasons:

Firstly, a wealth of research and clinical experience has shown that metformin can effectively eliminate abnormal cells, boost tissue regeneration, and adjust immune responses. This occurs through its ability to produce reactive oxygen species (ROS) at the cellular level, similar to the action seen in anti-tumor immune responses.

Secondly, using metformin off-label for non-diabetic conditions is both legally acceptable and generally safe.

Thirdly, metformin is well-tolerated by most individuals, with mild diarrhea being the most frequent side effect.

Additionally, metformin has been found to offer various health benefits, including weight loss, life extension, cancer inhibition, and anti-inflammatory effects. These serendipitous benefits are akin to those observed with chlorine dioxide. Unlike some targeted cancer therapies, which can lead to resistance, metformin can be safely used over a long period.

Lastly, metformin is a cost-effective option, enhancing its accessibility for broader use.

6. THE CANCER MODELS

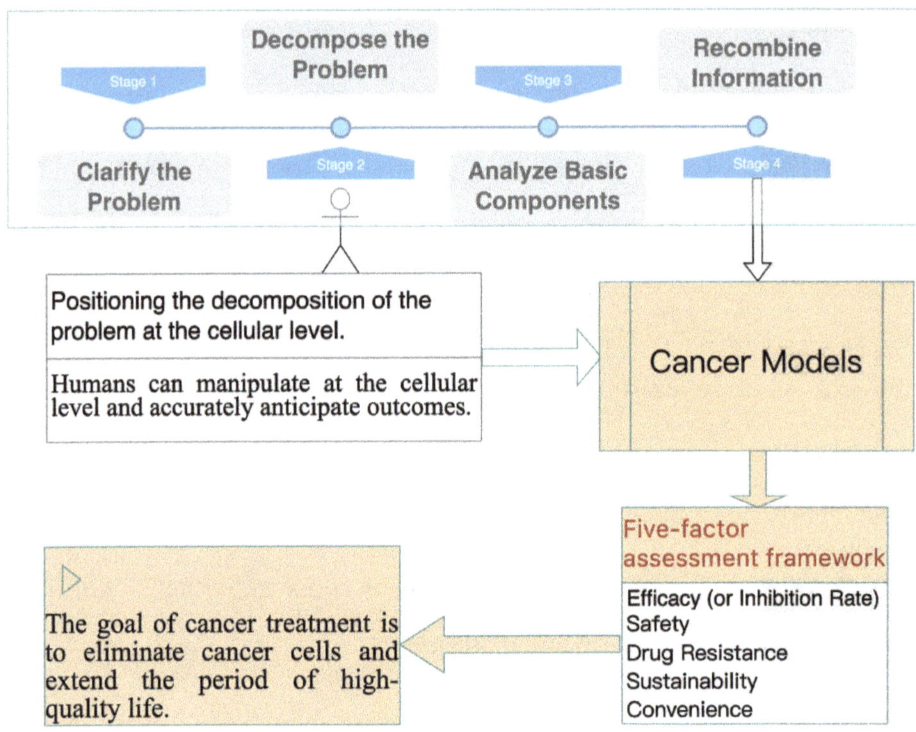

Using the logic of life models, we replace aging cells with cancer cells to construct a mathematical model. The total number of cancer cells is described by the following mathematical model:

$$V(t) = V_0 \frac{e^{k_1 t}}{(1 + k_2 t)^{\beta \frac{k_1}{k_2}}}$$

when the total number of cancer cells reaches a certain proportion (i.e., the proportion of cancer cells to the total number of cells in the body), the patient will die. The goal of our cancer treatment is to clear cancer cells more effectively, preventing their total number from reaching the lethal proportion[2].

A treatment method without side effects might follow the pattern described below. When a cancer therapy can directly eliminate some cancer cells without any side effects, the patient will live longer after this treatment. The extension of life is directly proportional to the percentage of cancer cells removed. Although this therapy has no side effects, meaning it does not weaken the immune system's ability to fight cancer, it also does not enhance it. After a short-term decrease in the total number of cancer cells, their count will eventually begin to increase again, following the previous pattern.

The diagram below models the treatment of cancer using a therapy known as CD cancer treatment. In this model, time is measured in days for mice and months for humans. A CD therapy is administered when the

---

[2] For readers with a mathematical background, you can explore the Further Reading section of this book, which contains the full content of the mathematical model of cancer.

tumor reaches a specific size, with a set point for when it becomes lethal. This treatment directly reduces the tumor size and enhances immune function. As a result, the tumor is reduced to 51% of its original size, effectively shifting the progression of the tumor earlier by several periods, which delays the advancement of the disease.

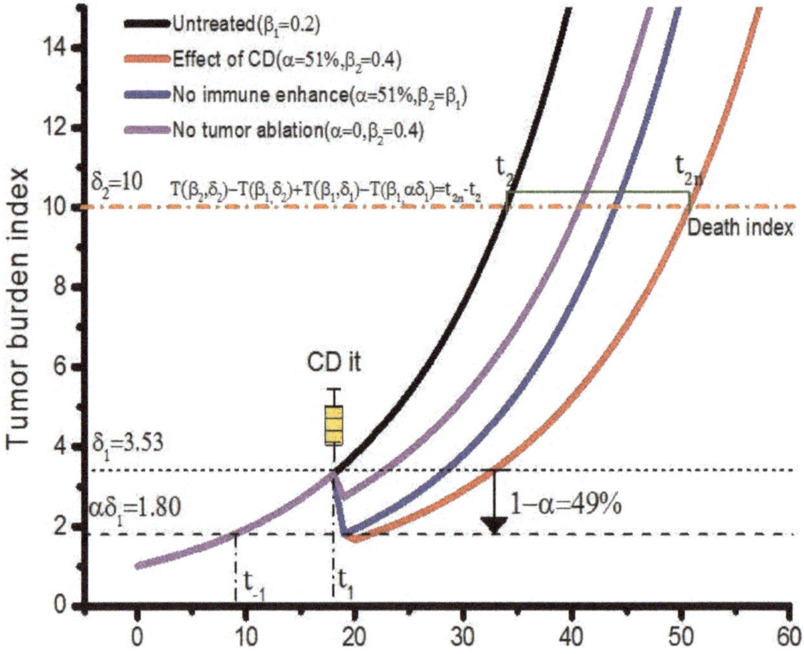

If a cancer treatment method can be used continuously and reapplied before the total number of cancer cells crosses the mortality threshold, ideally each treatment would also enhance the immune system's ability to eliminate cancer cells. Theoretically, this approach could extend a patient's life indefinitely, as illustrated in the figure below.

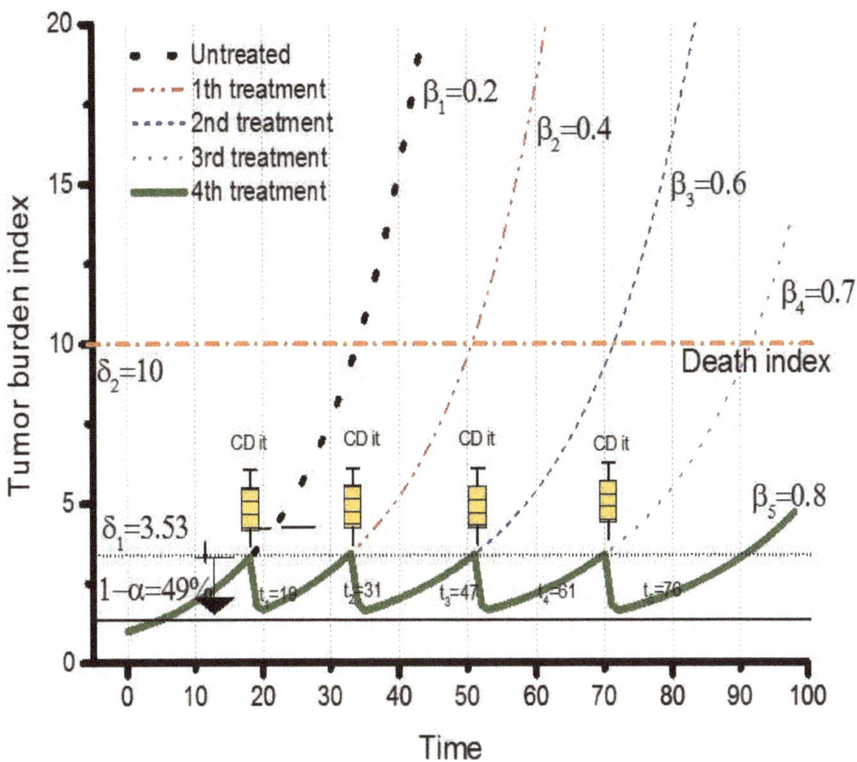

For a treatment to be sustainable, it must not lead to drug resistance. In the Further Reading section, we have refined our model to include variables for drug resistance. When a therapy develops resistance, the cancer treatment model undergoes significant changes. Simply eliminating cancer cells is not the best strategy; it is more effective to maintain sensitive cancer cells within a controlled range rather than completely killing them off. This is because cancer cells compete with each other, and eliminating all sensitive cells provides space and nutrients that accelerate the growth of resistant cells. This concept can be explained by the ecological dynamics in Siberia, where deer, wolves, and tigers coexist. Initially, hunting tigers to increase deer populations led to an increase in wolves and a decrease in deer. Later, banning tiger hunting allowed tiger populations to recover, which in turn decreased wolves and increased deer. When multiple competitors exist, eliminating one can inadvertently increase the others.

Even without mathematical models, we can deduce that resistance is a serious problem in cancer treatment, leading to unsustainable therapies and leaving patients in advanced stages without viable treatment options. Most current cancer therapies face some level of resistance. Research indicates that even physical methods like radiation therapy develop resistance. Targeted drugs are inherently resistant, as they are designed to attack cancer cells with specific mutations. Due to the heterogeneity of cancer, mutations are numerous, and targeted drugs can only kill a subset of sensitive cells, not the resistant ones. Even immunotherapies, such as PD-1 inhibitors, exhibit some resistance. Any therapy that selectively kills certain types of cancer cells is inherently prone to resistance and often cannot be used continuously.

While drug resistance is a major factor in the sustainability of cancer treatment, other factors also play a significant role. For example, surgery poses similar challenges to sustainability. It's clear that cancer surgeries, especially radical surgeries that remove entire organs, are difficult to repeat. Not only do these surgeries aim to remove all cancerous tissues, they often also remove some healthy tissue, making repeated surgeries less feasible.

Using cancer models, we can identify five key factors that are crucial for achieving the ultimate goals of cancer treatment. These factors are: efficacy(or inhibition rate), safety, resistance, sustainability, and convenience. Each of these plays a critical role in determining whether cancer treatment can be successful in the long term.

6.1 Efficacy (or Inhibition Rate)

Efficacy refers to the rate at which cancer cells are eliminated; a high efficacy indicates that the cancer treatment is highly effective at killing cancer cells. In cancer treatment, efficacy is the simplest and most common measure, and it is often the primary goal of almost all cancer therapies. Many new treatments even set efficacy as their sole target. A clinical trial can prove a treatment or new drug effective by achieving just one clinical endpoint, and efficacy is the easiest effect to observe in the short term. However, once a treatment or drug is approved, other critical variables like safety might be overlooked.

While a higher efficacy is always desirable, it should not be pursued at the expense of other attributes. Efficacy is crucial, but it is not everything.

In our life model, we discuss two pathways to clear senescent cells: one is direct elimination through specific therapies, and the other enhances the immune system's capability to naturally engage in the clearance process. Similarly, in our cancer model, there are two pathways to eliminate cancer cells: direct removal and activating the immune system to enhance its ability to clear cancer cells.

For cancer patients choosing a treatment plan, it's essential to consider the efficacy of the recommended therapies or drugs, which could stem from direct clearance, reliance on the immune system, or a combination of both. A treatment that offers both direct clearance capabilities and the ability to activate the immune system for a systemic elimination of cancer cells should be preferred. For example, surgical tumor removal typically only directly clears cancer cells and rarely boosts immune function. In contrast, many interventional ablation procedures not only directly ablate cancer cells but also release tumor antigens that enhance the immune system's anticancer capabilities. Given similar conditions, cancer patients should prefer interventional ablation procedures.

6.2 Safety

Safety in cancer treatment, particularly regarding the side effects of therapies, is crucial. While the threshold for tolerating side effects in developing cancer therapies is high, this does not imply that safety concerns can be overlooked. For cancer patients, side effects that are not life-threatening may seem minor compared to the prospect of death. However, since most cancer drugs fundamentally act as poisons due to their toxic properties, doctors often view side effects as an unavoidable consequence.

In many cases, cancer patients might overlook the side effects of their treatments. However, they may later discover side effects that severely impact their quality of life. For example, 80% of patients who undergo hysterectomy develop neurogenic bladder, a form of urinary incontinence, which in severe cases can lead to hydronephrosis and kidney failure. Annually, about 2.5 million hysterectomies are performed in China and approximately 400,000 in the United States. Most of these patients experience urinary system issues because radical surgeries aimed at removing all cancerous tissues can easily damage internal nerves.

Furthermore, nearly 100% of patients undergoing chemotherapy experience various side effects, with 80% suffering from severe anemia. The side effects of cancer treatment seem to be the cost of high efficacy, but it is crucial to recognize that most of these side effects damage the immune system, reducing or eliminating the body's natural anticancer immune capabilities, thus increasing the likelihood of cancer recurrence. Clearly, these side effects are not worth the trade-off, as the true goal for patients is not short-term cancer suppression, but a longer, healthier life. Sacrificing long-term benefits for short-term high efficacy by damaging the immune system is not justified.

The human immune system plays a continuous role in fighting cancer, even when cancer is present. The immune system is a natural anticancer tool, and if future treatments damage this system, the patient's future becomes bleaker, with short-term cancer suppression potentially shortening rather than extending life.

When choosing therapies for cancer patients, while it might be impossible to find treatments or drugs without any side effects, those with fewer side effects and higher safety should be prioritized. For instance, the side effects of chemotherapy drugs largely stem from their systemic application, spreading toxic substances throughout the body. I am aware of a private hospital in China, named after its founder Bofa Hospital, which has adopted a new method of drug delivery by injecting chemotherapy drugs directly into the tumor. This approach significantly reduces side effects while maintaining the desired inhibitory effects of chemotherapy, potentially offering higher efficacy than traditional methods.

6.3 Drug Resistance

While drug resistance differs from safety concerns, the outcomes can be similar. In the pursuit of high short-term suppression rates, clinical trials often limit their focus to a subset of patients with high mutations in specific targets, which almost invariably leads to drug resistance. We've discussed how overly complex technological solutions can lead to more problems before fully understanding the relationship between genetic mutations and cellular changes. Short-term fixes targeting genetic mutations can lead to more complex long-term issues. In applying first principles to complex problems, it's crucial to avoid falling into the trap of reductionism, which involves breaking down problems to an excessively detailed level. Since there's still much uncertainty below the cellular level, it's sufficient to break down the basic components of cancer treatment to the cellular level.

The medical research community often prides itself on using complex technologies, which inevitably lead to complex issues such as drug resistance. Unfortunately, cancer patients and doctors, who are guided by established guidelines, are often powerless to change this trend. However, as patients, we can choose treatments with lower or no resistance from the options provided by doctors.

The fundamental cause of drug resistance is that treatments or drugs selectively kill only those cancer cells sensitive to them. Once there are no sensitive cells left in the cancer tissue, the treatment or drug can no longer suppress the malignant proliferation of the cancer. Although cancer cells share certain characteristics, each cancer tissue is heterogeneous, characterized by hundreds of mutations. Targeting drugs that focus on a single mutation can only kill a subset of cancer cells. However, drugs like Gleevec have shown much better results for certain blood cancers with a singular mutation profile. Since its release in 2001, Gleevec has shown an effectiveness rate of over 94% in treating chronic myeloid leukemia, with 76% of patients returning to normal levels and ratios of various blood cells.

However, such cancers are not common, and most cancers, particularly solid tumors, are characterized by their heterogeneity and resistance to targeted drugs. While it might seem feasible to gradually develop targeted drugs for various mutations, it's not that simple. In our cancer models, we see that once a targeted drug develops resistance, it no longer suppresses resistant cancer cells. Instead, by eliminating competitive cancer cells, it allows resistant cells to proliferate more rapidly. Essentially, while the drug might reduce the size of the tumor in the short term, it actually shortens the patient's life. [3]

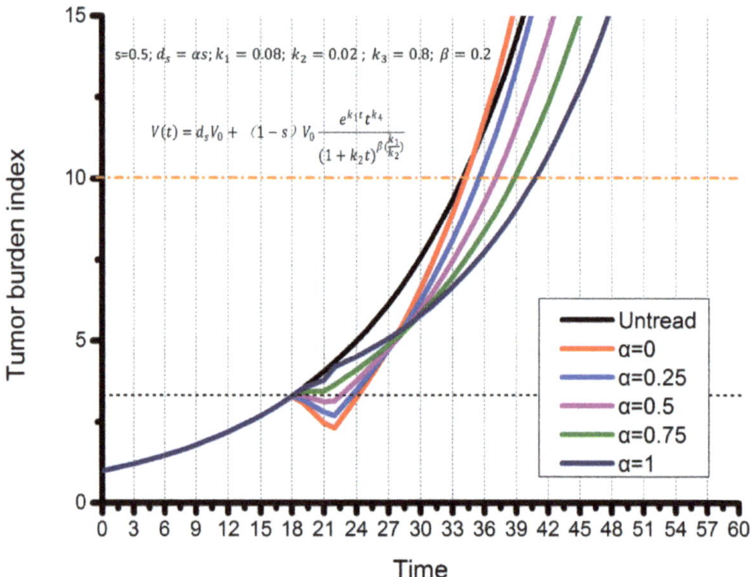

---

[3] The mathematical model shown in the figure below can be found in the Further Reading section. In this model, the initial tumor burden index (V_0) is set at 3.3 at the start of cancer treatment. When treatment begins with a drug that causes resistance, a higher dosage results in more significant tumor reduction but a shorter extension of the patient's expected survival time. Conversely, reducing the drug dosage to a level that only maintains the non-proliferation of sensitive cancer cells without shrinking them results in a longer expected survival time. This model applies to a scenario where the proportion of drug-sensitive cancer cells is low, with ($s = 0.5$).

Similar to how some side effects merely reduce the quality of life while others can hasten death, drug resistance can paradoxically shorten life if targeted drugs effectively reduce tumor size in the short term but ultimately fail to extend the patient's life. This contradicts the ultimate goal of cancer treatment. Without applying first principles, such outcomes might become the norm, as both patients and doctors favor using complex, newly developed targeted and immunotherapeutic drugs.

By applying first principles, we would be particularly cautious in using drugs developed through complex molecular biology technologies. We should focus on the cellular level to use these drugs wisely and minimize their resistance, perhaps by maintaining a controlled number of sensitive cancer cells rather than eliminating them all, which can also suppress the proliferation of resistant cells. Additionally, we should reevaluate our models of cancer progression to consider both suppression rates and resistance, balancing short-term effects with long-term benefits and choosing treatments with a lower incidence of resistance.

6.4 Sustainability

Safety and drug resistance are major factors contributing to the unsustainability of cancer treatments. If the side effects of a cancer treatment are severe enough, they may prematurely end a patient's life; similarly, using the latest drug-resistant treatment methods might also shorten a patient's lifespan. Once a patient has passed away or is near death, not only is the treatment they were using no longer viable, but they are also unable to choose other cancer treatment options. Thus, we define the sustainability of cancer treatment as the ability to continue using a treatment method that consistently kills cancer cells, keeps the cancer burden below a lethal threshold, and extends the patient's life. Clearly, the sustainability of cancer treatment is a crucial component of cancer treatment goals and is indispensable.

Safety and drug resistance directly impact the sustainability of cancer treatments, which is easy to understand. However, there are also sustainable factors that are neither related to safety nor resistance but still affect the sustainability of cancer treatments. For example, surgical removal of cancer, which has almost no sustainability. If cancer is detected early and the lesion is relatively small, doctors generally recommend surgical removal. In the real medical environment, doctors tend to remove a larger portion of normal tissue to ensure that the cancer is completely excised. Surgical procedures are unlikely to stimulate the immune system to engage in anti-cancer activities, and without an enhanced immune system, the likelihood of cancer recurrence is high, regardless of whether there are residual cancer cells. Facing recurrent cancer, it is almost impossible for patients to undergo the same surgical removal again.

In cancer models, early detection and treatment indeed can increase patient survival, but this is under the assumption that there are no side effects or resistance. It is generally believed that small cancer surgeries effectively remove cancerous tissues without side effects or resistance. Therefore, guidelines advocating for early detection and treatment are based on the suitability of surgical removal for early-detected cancers. However, even if the sustainability of surgery is low, early detection and treatment do not necessarily benefit patients in the long term, and the extended survival period from early detection and treatment may not be as beneficial as other cancer treatments that are not based on early detection.

Understanding this perspective, let's consider a scenario: if a cancer patient misses the opportunity for early detection and surgical treatment, and the cancer is discovered too late for surgery, the patient can still choose other treatments similar to surgery, such as local tumor ablation. Local tumor ablation can not only kill the entire cancerous tissue like surgery but also has a proven benefit of stimulating the immune system's systemic anti-tumor capabilities.

When choosing a cancer treatment, patients must give considerable importance to the future sustainability of cancer treatments. In approved cancer treatments or when choosing better options from the NCCN guidelines, patients can still select sustainable cancer treatments based on our cancer model's systemic thinking (i.e., first principles).

6.5 Convenience

In the healthcare system, while convenience may not be as critical as other factors, it significantly influences patients' choices. Patients are likely to opt for more convenient treatments if other conditions are similar. Generally, convenience implies cost-effectiveness and sustainability. Once cancer patients enter a hospital, it must be acknowledged that most hospitals are motivated to recommend the latest and most expensive cancer treatments, often overlooking convenience in their decision-making. Even under guidelines that promote early detection and treatment, patients are typically advised to undergo complex surgeries rather than more convenient minimally invasive ablations. This is because a hospital may not be proficient in all cancer treatments and tends to adopt the latest and most complex technologies. Additionally, convenience is often associated with lower cost and perceived lower quality. For instance, In China, the cost of a cancer surgery is around $10,000, whereas the same tumor treated with radiofrequency ablation costs about $5,000. Local ablation procedures have fewer side effects and better immune activation compared to surgical excisions. Despite this, the number of patients choosing surgery significantly exceeds those opting for radiofrequency ablation.

Of course, the issue of convenience is less critical than other factors, and as technology advances, many cutting-edge techniques are making cancer treatments more convenient. For example, advancements in modern imaging equipment like CT, ultrasound, and MRI have simplified previously complex cancer treatments. Moreover, choosing convenient treatments does not necessarily mean sacrificing other metrics. While most oral medications are less effective than intravenous drugs, technological advancements have enabled highly effective treatments that offer convenience comparable to, or even better than, traditional methods. For instance, traditional radiotherapy has evolved into more effective proton or heavy ion therapy, and treatments that involve directly inserting radioactive materials into tumors are more convenient and as safe as proton therapy.

In summary, while convenience might limit some effective cancer treatments, the essence of first principles is to simplify complex problems. When applying first principles, convenience should not be considered in isolation but integrated with other metrics to make informed decisions about cancer treatment options. Particularly, decisions based solely on convenience are likely not optimal as its correlation with other important factors might be weak.

PART THREE: NAVIGATE YOUR CANCER JOURNEY

"Science is a way of thinking much more than it is a body of knowledge."

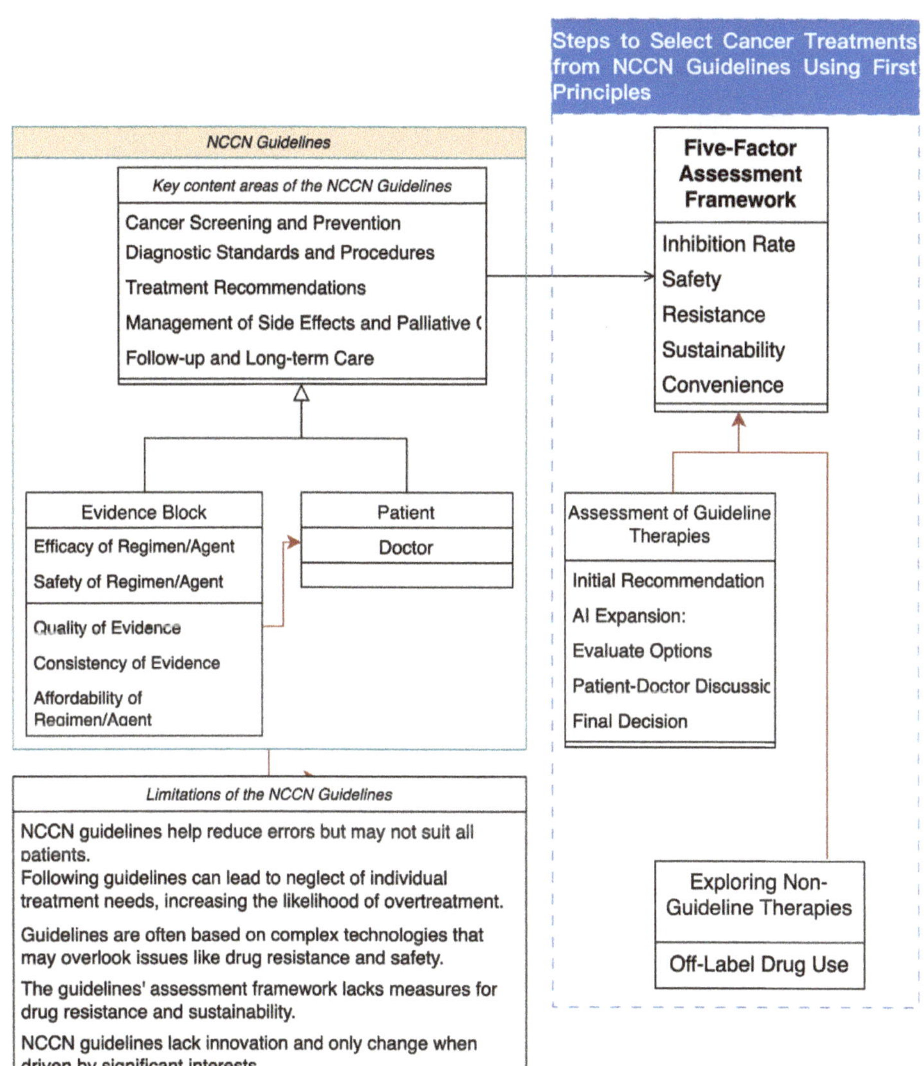

Steps to Select Cancer Treatments from NCCN Guidelines Using First Principles
NCCN Guidelines
Key content areas of the NCCN Guidelines
Cancer Screening and Prevention
Diagnostic Standards and Procedures
Treatment Recommendations
Management of Side Effects and Palliative (
Follow-up and Long-term Care
Five-Factor Assessment Framework
Inhibition Rate
Safety
Resistance
Sustainability
Convenience
Evidence Block
Efficacy of Regimen/Agent
Safety of Regimen/Agent
Quality of Evidence
Consistency of Evidence
Affordability of Regimen/Agent
Patient
Doctor
Assessment of Guideline Therapies
Initial Recommendation
AI Expansion:
Evaluate Options
Patient-Doctor Discussic
Final Decision
Limitations of the NCCN Guidelines
NCCN guidelines help reduce errors but may not suit all patients.
Following guidelines can lead to neglect of individual treatment needs, increasing the likelihood of overtreatment.
Guidelines are often based on complex technologies that may overlook issues like drug resistance and safety.
The guidelines' assessment framework lacks measures for drug resistance and sustainability.
NCCN guidelines lack innovation and only change when driven by significant interests.
Exploring Non-Guideline Therapies
Off-Label Drug Use

The National Comprehensive Cancer Network (NCCN), a nonprofit academic consortium made up of 21 leading cancer centers in the United States, publishes annual clinical practice guidelines for various malignancies that are recognized and followed by clinicians worldwide. The NCCN aims to enhance the quality of oncology services globally and benefit cancer patients. Dedicated to defining and advancing high-quality, high-value, patient-centered cancer care worldwide, the NCCN guidelines are acknowledged as the clinical direction and policy standard for cancer management. They are the most comprehensive and frequently updated clinical practice guidelines available across all medical fields. These guidelines are authored by multidisciplinary expert panels from 30 leading cancer centers in the U.S. Currently, there are 24 adapted versions and 230 translations of the NCCN guidelines, covering 47 different languages.

7.1 Content of the NCCN Guidelines

The NCCN Guidelines, developed by the National Comprehensive Cancer Network, are comprehensive, evidence-based clinical practice guidelines designed to standardize treatment pathways for cancer care. These guidelines encompass the entire continuum of cancer care, from prevention and diagnosis to treatment, follow-up, and palliative care, and are considered among the most authoritative and influential in global cancer treatment.

The guidelines are the collaborative work of multidisciplinary teams from top U.S. cancer centers, including oncologists, radiation specialists, surgeons, pathologists, nurses, and other relevant professionals. They are based on the latest scientific evidence and clinical trial results, and are regularly updated to reflect new research findings and advancements in treatment technologies.

Key content areas of the NCCN Guidelines include:

1) **Cancer Screening and Prevention:** The guidelines provide detailed information on risk assessment, screening, and prevention strategies for various cancers, including recommended screening schedules, methods, and preventive measures.

2) **Diagnostic** Standards **and Procedures:** They outline the diagnostic criteria and recommended diagnostic processes for various cancers, including necessary lab tests and imaging studies.

3) **Treatment Recommendations:** This core section offers detailed treatment plans for each type of cancer based on different clinical scenarios, including surgery, radiation therapy, chemotherapy, targeted therapy, and immunotherapy.

4) **Management of Side Effects and Palliative Care:** The guidelines also cover how to manage side effects during treatment and effective palliative care strategies to improve patients' quality of life.

5) **Follow-up and Long-term Care:** They provide recommendations for post-treatment follow-up strategies and long-term care to detect recurrences or metastases early and manage long-term complications of treatment.

The NCCN Guidelines are widely used in clinical practice to help healthcare providers make evidence-based treatment decisions. They also serve as a vital resource for educating and training healthcare professionals. In healthcare insurance and policy-making, the guidelines are often used as a standard for treatment coverage and reimbursement.

In summary, the NCCN Guidelines are a comprehensive, multidisciplinary, and evidence-based resource that provides detailed guidance on all aspects of cancer care. They are an indispensable tool for healthcare providers, researchers, and policymakers worldwide. The guidelines include all the latest approved therapies, and due to the advanced state of cancer research and high treatment costs in the U.S., they serve as a global clinical guide for cancer treatment applicable to patients in any country. While many countries have their own clinical practice guidelines for cancer, none are as comprehensive as the NCCN's, making it an essential toolkit for any cancer patient choosing treatment methods.

Doctors and patients can easily download and read the guidelines, which theoretically provide recommended therapies for any type of cancer. The NCCN guidelines feature an "Evidence Block" rating system that includes five indicators to comprehensively assess the overall value of a cancer treatment:

1) **Efficacy of Regimen/Agent**:

   o 5 points: Highly effective, potential for cure, usually offers long-term survival benefits.
   o 4 points: Very effective, though cure is less likely, can sometimes offer long-term survival benefits.
   o 3 points: Moderately effective, moderate impact on survival, often controls the disease.

- o 2 points: Minimally effective, no or unknown impact on survival, but can sometimes control the disease.
- o 1 point: Provides only symptom relief.

2) **Safety of Regimen/Agent**:

- o 5 points: Generally non-toxic, rare or minor toxicity, does not impact daily activities (ADLs).
- o 4 points: Occasional toxicity, significant toxicity is rare or only low-grade, minor impact on ADLs.
- o 3 points: Mild toxicity, interferes with ADLs.
- o 2 points: Moderate toxicity, frequently significant but non-life-threatening/fatal toxicity; often interferes with ADLs.
- o 1 point: Highly toxic, frequently significant or life-threatening/fatal toxicity; usually severely interferes with ADLs.

3) **Quality of Evidence**:

- o 5 points: High quality, multiple well-designed randomized trials and/or meta-analyses.
- o 4 points: Good quality, one or more well-designed randomized trials.
- o 3 points: Average quality, low-quality randomized trials or well-designed non-randomized trials.
- o 2 points: Low quality, case reports or extensive clinical experience.
- o 1 point: Poor quality, little to no evidence.

4) **Consistency of Evidence**:

- o 5 points: Highly consistent, multiple trials with similar results.
- o 4 points: Mostly consistent, some variability in results across multiple trials.

- o 3 points: Possibly consistent, few trials or trials with few patients, whether randomized or not, some variability in results.
- o 2 points: Inconsistent, clear differences in the direction of results between quality trials.
- o 1 point: Anecdotal evidence, based on human anecdotal experiences.

5) **Affordability of Regimen/Agent** (including drug costs, supportive care, infusions, toxicity monitoring, and toxicity management):

- o 5 points: Very inexpensive.
- o 4 points: Inexpensive.
- o 3 points: Moderately expensive.
- o 2 points: Expensive.
- o 1 point: Very expensive.

These indicators help healthcare professionals comprehensively evaluate the benefits of cancer treatment options, including efficacy, safety, quality of evidence, consistency of evidence, and cost-effectiveness, thereby providing patients with the best treatment choices.

7.2 Limitations of the NCCN Guidelines

While the NCCN guidelines encompass all cancer types and their respective treatments, guiding doctors in choosing specific treatment plans for individual cancer patients, they are somewhat akin to a mobile map app, marking all locations and routes on a map. For a specific cancer patient, there are many navigational routes, and doctors need to select the best navigation based on their expertise. In other words, there are many treatment methods, and which one benefits a cancer patient depends entirely on the decisions of the doctor and the patient.

Our previous chapters have shown that the overall level of cancer treatment has become more unified due to the guidelines, and it seems to have improved in the short term. However, in the long term, the level of treatment has not significantly improved due to this standardized treatment guideline. On the contrary, the guidelines have somewhat oversimplified cancer treatment. While standardized treatment reduces errors and benefits some patients, it may also harm others who should not be treated according to the guideline.

Guidelines can standardize cancer treatment, and even if the treatment methods recommended by the guidelines benefit everyone without considering individual differences, this could promote overtreatment. Since doctors can avoid liability by simply following the guidelines, without considering the safety, drug resistance, and sustainability of the chosen cancer therapy, doctors around the world might overtreat patients.

All content in the guidelines is supported by clinical research, but as we have discussed before, medicine tends to pursue complex technologies at the molecular level, often creating more problems than solutions, such as drug resistance and safety issues. The guidelines, without comparison, regularly update to include cancer treatment technologies that focus only on short-term benefits, potentially extending a patient's life by just three months in more than 50% of the treatments.

The field of research publication rarely includes studies with negative effects, hence there is a lack of scrutiny of the negative aspects of existing cancer therapies in the entire medical research community. A cancer drug with significant long-term side effects may remain in the guidelines for a long time because the guidelines are set by authorities in the field, and who would challenge such authority, even though these academic authorities are essentially performing the work of an intelligent search robot.

Although the guidelines provide a five-factor framework for assessing the comprehensive value of cancer treatments, comparing it to the five-factor framework based on first principles proposed in this book reveals its lack of comprehensiveness. Specifically, the five-factor assessment framework in the guidelines includes the inhibition rate (corresponding to the "efficacy" indicator in the guidelines), safety (corresponding to the "safety" indicator), and convenience (corresponding to the "affordability" indicator). However, for factors that particularly affect the long-term interests of patients, such as drug resistance and sustainability, there are no corresponding indicators in the guidelines. This situation reflects the broader context of the existing medical system and medical research, where these two factors are often overlooked. Moreover, most treatments in the guidelines, especially new treatments or drugs added during annual updates, usually perform poorly in these two areas.

The NCCN guidelines are akin to the rocket launches before SpaceX, where countries under NASA's influence were advancing launch technology, but no innovator in the industry proposed reusable rockets. Similar to the cancer treatment field's NCCN guidelines, NASA also has an advanced launch manual, and other countries follow this standard, whether intentionally or not, with no one in the industry motivated to break with tradition. It was only when Musk, who values cost-effectiveness, proposed and led SpaceX to develop reusable rockets that people realized that only when major interests of the parties involved are at stake will the motivation to break with tradition appear. However, breaking with authoritative guidelines in the cancer treatment field is unimaginable, facing far greater obstacles than rocket launching. This book does not advise patients to seek cancer treatments beyond the guidelines; instead, it guides cancer patients to influence their doctors with first principles during discussions and choose the most beneficial cancer treatment plan according to the guidelines.

7.3 Steps for Selecting Existing Cancer Treatments in the NCCN Guidelines Using First Principles

In previous chapters, we've clarified two key conditions for applying first principles in cancer treatment. The first condition involves focusing treatment operations at the cellular level, where we can directly manipulate and anticipate outcomes using modern therapeutic means. The second condition is that the objectives of cancer treatment should be set according to our cancer model, aiming to eradicate cancer cells and enable patients to maintain a high quality of life. Under these conditions, we incorporate five observable variables into our model: inhibition rate, safety, drug resistance, sustainability, and convenience. By evaluating each treatment's performance on these variables, we determine its ability to control the long-term burden of cancer, thus allowing us to score each treatment comprehensively. Treatments with higher scores are prioritized.

Step one. After a cancer patient is diagnosed, they usually receive treatment recommendations from their doctor based on the NCCN guidelines. Depending on the type and stage of cancer, the guidelines may offer up to ten treatment options for the doctor to choose from, and the doctor will typically recommend about two options for the patient to consider. Often, patients find it challenging to choose from the options provided by their doctor and may end up selecting the treatment recommended by the doctor.

Step two. According to first principles, we should not blindly follow the choices outlined in the guidelines. With existing artificial intelligence and data processing tools, patients can actually select more treatment options from the guidelines, especially those applicable to different stages or types of tumors. The main purpose of this approach is to find the most suitable treatment option from a broader range, as a patient's specific cancer characteristics may not fully match the descriptions in the standard treatment guidelines. I am developing an AI tool for selecting cancer treatment options that combines large language models with first principles. This tool will be able to choose treatments that go beyond the recommendations of the NCCN guidelines, with the preliminary idea being that this AI tool could provide twice as many alternative options as those recommended by the guidelines. Although this increases the complexity of choice and may overwhelm some patients, the expansion is almost instantaneous with the help of AI tools, and we believe there is a high likelihood of finding treatment options that better align with first principles.

Step three. Choosing from up to twenty treatment options is a crucial step in decision-making using first principles. Patients should evaluate these treatment options based on scores in inhibition rate, safety, drug resistance, sustainability, and convenience. Initially, each indicator can be given equal weight, and their weighted average score can be calculated. The treatment option with the highest score should be the one chosen by the patient. For example, an intratumoral injection therapy for a specific solid tumor received a score of 86 out of 100 in a simulated rating table for these five factors, indicating that this therapy is a suitable treatment method for that particular solid tumor.

Cancer Treatment Scoring Chart

Key Dimensions	Scores (out of 100)	The Reasons for the Scores.	Causes of Losing Points
Convenience	50	With the advancement of puncture techniques, intra-tumor injection is becoming increasingly easier.	It is less convenient than oral and intravenous injection.
Safety	95	The greatest advantage of intra-tumor injection is the absence of	Inevitably, it causes some damage to normal tissues.

		systemic side effects.	
Inhibition Rate	90	Multiple pathways to inhibit injected tumors.	The inhibitory rate for tumors not injected remains relatively low.
Drug Resistance	100	Kills cancer cells without selection, eliminating drug resistance.	
Sustainability	95	It can be used repeatedly for long-term sustainability.	The convenience of intratumoral injection is relatively low.
Average Score	86		

Step four. In the steps described above, patients have completed significant preparatory work by researching and selecting treatment options on their own. I believe most doctors would appreciate this approach. Once patients have identified the best treatment plan, they can confidently discuss it with their doctor. Since the first principles approach employs fundamental human reasoning, doctors can fully understand when patients present their selection process, especially the evaluation method of the five factors. On one hand, the patient's choice aligns with the guidelines' recommended methods; on the other hand, doctors usually possess more medical knowledge than patients, so they find it easier to understand and accept decisions that are logical and based on first principles.

Step five. Treatment proceeds with the selected plan if both doctor and patient agree. It's important to note that the treatment plan chosen based on first principles might not always be the best option recommended in the guidelines, or even the one initially suggested by the doctor. However, we must trust that as the most important stakeholders and direct beneficiaries of the treatment plan, patients have a deep understanding of their own treatment options. This understanding can help them overcome inherent fears and hesitations. By being more proactive and involved in the treatment process, patients may achieve better treatment outcomes and quality of life.

7.4 The Helsinki Declaration and Off-Label Drug Use

The Helsinki Declaration, primarily aimed at clinical research and trials involving human subjects, also offers guidelines for the use of unproven treatments in clinical practice. These guidelines help doctors provide potential treatment opportunities ethically when no other effective options are known.

Specifically, the Declaration includes guidance on individual medical actions, particularly in its section on "unproven interventions." It states that, in the absence of standard interventions or after these have been exhausted, doctors may use unproven interventions with the informed consent of the patient or their legal representative, provided these measures are likely to save life, restore health, or alleviate suffering. This is based on the professional judgment of the doctor and usually under the advice of experts.

This part of the Declaration reflects a comprehensive consideration of medical ethics, extending beyond the scope of clinical trials to everyday medical practice. This helps ensure the protection of patient rights while also promoting the exploration and use of new treatments by doctors under ethical principles.

SpaceX has disrupted traditional rocket launch models by successfully developing reusable rockets, significantly reducing costs and increasing the scale of spacecraft launches. Similarly, while traditional cancer treatment models are hard to break, we can choose uncommon but potentially more suitable treatments for cancer patients' long-term goals within the existing medical system. For example, unproven interventions represent a chance to break away from traditional cancer treatment models using individual initiative. When a patient feels that existing cancer treatments are ineffective, they should also have the capability to explore unproven interventions. In large hospitals, various factors, especially professional risks, make it difficult for doctors to adopt unproven interventions; however, in smaller hospitals, there may be more opportunities to implement such treatments.

The most common form of unproven intervention is likely the off-label use of drugs. In the current medical system, completely unproven interventions are rare. In reality, some small hospitals openly specialize in off-label treatments for cancer patients. For instance, in China, a renowned professor named Baofa established three small hospitals named Baofa

Hospitals in Shandong and Beijing, which openly promote a cancer treatment method involving intratumoral injection of chemotherapy drugs, attracting thousands of treatment cases from multiple countries. Intratumoral injection of chemotherapy drugs is an interesting idea to reduce the systemic side effects of chemotherapy drugs without sacrificing their inhibitory rate. Additionally, the resistance to chemotherapy drugs and the sustainability of intratumoral injections are good treatment ideas, and the convenience has significantly improved with medical technology advancements. The biggest challenge with intratumoral injection of chemotherapy drugs is how to keep the drugs in the tumor long enough to maximize their cytotoxic effects on cancer cells. According to Baofa Hospitals, they use a slow-release technology to affect the action of chemotherapy drugs.

In the United States, similar small hospitals are dedicated to an off-label use of anticancer drugs. Williams Cancer Institute, with three cancer centers in Mexico and the United States, uses a combination therapy of tumor ablation and intratumoral injection of immunotherapy drugs to treat cancer patients. Previously, immunotherapy drugs like PD-1 needed to be administered intravenously, which would distribute throughout the body. However, by combining tumor ablation technology with direct injection of immunotherapy drugs into the tumor, it is said to enhance the effect of the immunotherapy drugs. Tumor ablation releases antigens, and combined with immunotherapy drugs, it can increase the inhibition rate while reducing costs, as PD-1 drugs are particularly expensive and their systemic use could be wasteful.

Based on our cancer model, the off-label treatment approaches of these two hospitals maximize the long-term effects of existing cancer drugs, aligning well with our first principles. There might be many other small hospitals adopting various unproven interventions, and with today's advanced information, cancer patients who have learned our first principles of cancer treatment can easily discover such new therapies.

Just as in selecting the best therapy methods in the NCCN guidelines, under the protection of the Helsinki Declaration, cancer patients can incorporate these off-label treatment methods into their options. Using a five-factor scoring method, all options are evaluated together, and the cancer treatment plan with the highest weighted average score is selected. If the final choice is an off-label treatment method, one must first reject the original doctor and proceed alone to a small private hospital for treatment. Since visiting a private small hospital might not be covered by insurance, this factor needs to be incorporated into the five-factor evaluation method and may require reassessment. For example, in the United States, the cost of cancer treatment not covered by medical insurance could reach as high as $100,000. Conversely, if choosing to undergo off-label drug treatment at a hospital in China, the expense might be only $10,000.

8. USING FIRST PRINCIPLES TO DECIDE ON CANCER TREATMENT OPTIONS

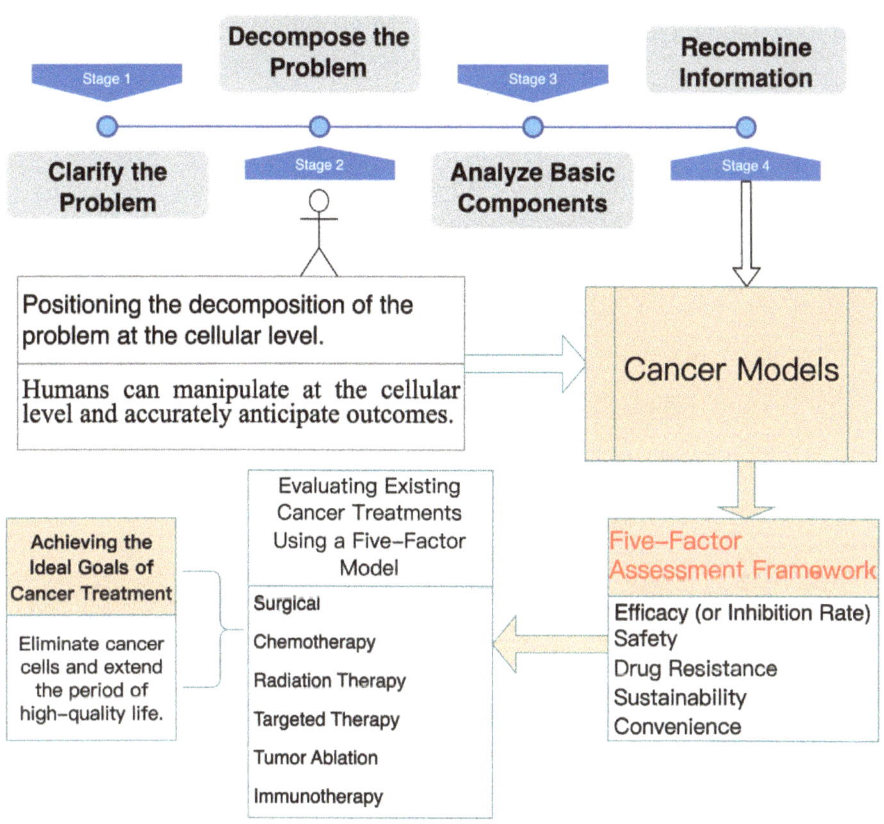

8.1 Building a Cancer Treatment Analysis Model Using First Principles

In the previous chapter, we established a mathematical model transitioning from a life model to a cancer model, completing the fourth step of the first principles approach. Now, we will detail the process of building a cancer treatment analysis model using first principles.

We begin by defining the problem, specifically how to effectively treat cancer while maximizing the protection of healthy cells. Next, we break down the problem to the cellular level, which not only deepens our understanding of cancer's cellular mechanisms but also helps address the reductionist tendencies in medical research.

We then analyze these fundamental components—the biological characteristics of cancerous and healthy cells and their responses under different treatment methods. Using this information, we apply basic biological and physical laws to construct a mathematical model that simulates the impact of various treatments on cancer and healthy cells.

Finally, we recombine this information to build a comprehensive cancer treatment analysis model. This model is not only based on our in-depth understanding at the cellular level but also integrates multiple assessments of treatment effects, such as inhibition rate, safety, resistance, sustainability, and convenience. This provides a holistic framework to help doctors and patients choose the most suitable treatment options and guides researchers in developing new methods.

Here is a breakdown of the process:

1) **Clarify the True Problem**: We must thoroughly understand the nature of cancer—a disease defined by the uncontrolled growth and spread of abnormal cells. The key to treating cancer lies in eradicating these malignant cells, halting their proliferation and spread, while preserving healthy cells as much as possible, ultimately aiming to prolong the patient's life with quality.

2) **Decompose the Problem**: Identifying the problem seems **straightforward**—find the most effective way to eliminate cancer cells while protecting healthy cells. However, a deeper analysis of this problem requires a more comprehensive approach. Analyzing the basic components at the cellular level is key to introducing the first principles approach to solving cancer treatment issues. This also helps correct the reductionist tendencies in medical research.

3) **Analyze Basic Components**: The current level of cancer treatment is not high, and it's challenging to develop new plans based on existing **research**. Doctors may not always choose the most patient-beneficial approach, and overtreatment is a serious issue. Existing treatment plans are often not the best solution for the cancer problem. Starting from first principles, we break down the problem, start with the most basic components, use basic laws to build an analysis model, and find the real answer to the problem.

4) **Recombine Information**: In this step, we used the second law of thermodynamics at the cellular level to build a life model, defining disordered **cells** as aging cells and viewing the accumulation of aging cells as the aging process. By analyzing the relationship between cancer and aging, we view cancer as part of aging. Using this life model, we constructed a cancer model that adheres to first principles. Through this model, we clarified the key issues in solving cancer treatment, aiming to achieve the goal of long-term high-

quality life for cancer patients, which requires excellent performance in the five variables of inhibition rate, safety, resistance, sustainability, and convenience.

We can represent the steps outlined above in a flowchart as follows:

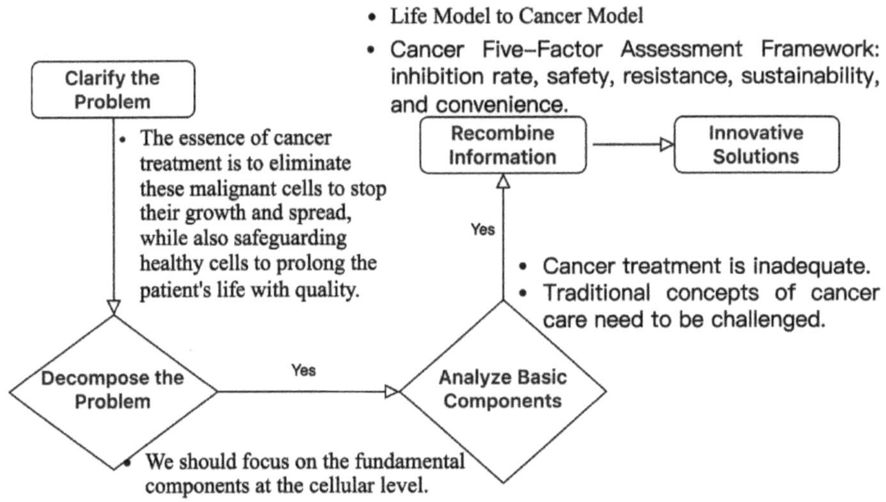

8.2 Evaluating Existing Cancer Treatments Using a Five-Factor Framework

Using the first principles-based cancer treatment analysis model, we've identified five key factors that significantly impact the ultimate goal of cancer treatment: extending the patient's high-quality survival period. This new assessment method allows us to reevaluate existing cancer treatment methods to ensure that treatments extend not just the survival period but the high-quality survival period of patients. This evaluation considers the long-term effects of treatment rather than just short-term outcomes.

Now, we can use this new assessment framework to provide truly meaningful treatment choices for individual patients. The advantage of this method is that it does not conflict with the existing medical system, as the chosen treatment plans are still those recommended in the NCCN guidelines. Thus, cancer patients can truly participate in the decision-making process of their treatment plans, and this involvement is more beneficial for doctors to provide personalized treatment.

To further guide cancer patients in applying this set of ideas during the cancer-fighting process, we will conduct a detailed analysis and evaluation of the following six common treatment plans. Through a comprehensive analysis of these treatment plans, cancer patients can obtain detailed information about each treatment method, including their advantages, limitations, and applicable conditions. This information will help patients and doctors make joint decisions, choosing the treatment plan that best fits their condition characteristics and quality of life requirements.

The application of this assessment method not only makes the treatment process more transparent but also enhances patient autonomy, allowing them to participate in treatment decisions based on their specific situations and preferences. This personalized treatment strategy will ultimately be more beneficial for the long-term health and quality of life of patients.

1. Cancer Surgery

Surgical treatment is a common method for addressing cancer, primarily aimed at removing tumors and potential cancer cells to reduce or eliminate the disease within the patient's body. The type, scope, and complexity of the surgery vary depending on the type, location, stage of the cancer, and the patient's overall health. Common surgical approaches include excision, which involves removing the tumor and some surrounding normal tissue, and radical surgery, which aims to completely remove the source of the cancer and associated lymph nodes.

Pre-surgical preparation includes a comprehensive physical examination, blood tests, and imaging studies to assess the patient's health status and surgical risks. Doctors discuss the potential risks and expected outcomes with patients to ensure they fully understand the necessity and possible consequences of the surgery. Surgery is usually performed under general anesthesia, and surgeons, depending on the type and purpose of the surgery, precisely remove the tumor and potentially affected surrounding tissues. High-precision tools like microscopes and endoscopes may be used to enhance the accuracy and safety of the procedure.

During the post-surgery recovery period, patients may need to stay in the hospital for observation. Doctors closely monitor the patient's recovery and potential complications, which may include pain management, wound care, and physical therapy. Like all surgeries, cancer surgery carries certain risks and potential complications, such as infection, bleeding, anesthesia-related risks, and long-term physiological or psychological effects. Doctors assess these risks based on the patient's specific conditions and take appropriate preventive measures.

If the cancer is in an early stage, surgical treatment often dominates due to its ability to remove all visible tumor tissue at once, achieving the highest rate of suppression. In the short term, because of its direct and rapid effects, surgical treatment is often the easiest option for patients to accept.

Following the principle of "early detection, early treatment," doctors and patients usually prefer surgical treatment; however, if the cancer has progressed to an intermediate stage, the conventional approach is to first use chemotherapy or targeted drugs to shrink the tumor, followed by surgical removal. The table below evaluates general cancer surgical treatments based on five factors.

Cancer Surgery Scorecard

Key Dimensions	Scores (out of 100)	The Reasons for the Scores.	Causes of Losing Points
Inhibition Rate	100	Removing tumor tissue has an immediate effect.	
Safety	50	The procedure is relatively safe.	Postoperative complications are common, and the unavoidable removal of normal tissue can impair its function.

Drug Resistance	100	There is no resistance to the treatment.	
Sustainability	10	If there are only a few recurrent tumors, surgery is still an option.	In most cases, it is difficult to operate again on the primary and metastatic sites.
Convenience	30	Surgical procedures are standardized, and any skilled surgeon can perform them.	Surgery remains a complex treatment method, and intraoperative risks need to be managed.
Average Score	58		

2. Chemotherapy

Chemotherapy is a common method for treating cancer, utilizing chemical drugs to attack and destroy cancer cells. These drugs can block the growth and division of cancer cells, helping to shrink tumors, control the spread of the disease, or alleviate symptoms. Chemotherapy can be used alone or in combination with surgery, radiation, or other treatments to enhance its effectiveness.

There is a wide variety of chemotherapy drugs, each with its specific mechanism of action. Some drugs may damage the DNA of cancer cells, preventing them from replicating and growing; others may interfere with specific proteins or signaling pathways that cancer cells use to grow. Doctors select the most appropriate drug or combination of drugs based on the patient's condition and type of cancer.

Chemotherapy can be administered in various ways, including orally, by intravenous injection, or directly into body cavities like the cerebrospinal fluid. The frequency and duration of treatment depend on the specific drugs and the treatment plan, which could be daily, weekly, or monthly.

Despite its key role in controlling cancer, chemotherapy can cause a range of side effects. These are primarily due to the fact that chemotherapy drugs affect not only cancer cells but also normal cells that divide rapidly, such as blood cells, cells in the digestive tract, and hair follicle cells. Common side effects include hair loss, nausea, vomiting, fatigue, loss of appetite, and mouth sores. The severity of these side effects varies from person to person, and many can be managed with medication and other treatment approaches.

During chemotherapy, patients need regular blood tests and other physical examinations to monitor their body's response to the treatment. This monitoring helps in timely adjusting the treatment plan to address potential complications or side effects, ensuring the safety and effectiveness of the treatment. Overall, chemotherapy is a complex process that requires close cooperation and coordination among doctors, patients, and their families to achieve the best treatment outcomes and quality of life.

Compared to surgical treatment, the inhibitory effects of chemotherapy are generally lower, and it is associated with more side effects. This is mainly because chemotherapy drugs are not delivered directly to the tumor tissue but are administered systemically. Since the tumor tissue constitutes only a small part of the body, the effective concentration of chemotherapy drugs at the tumor site is significantly reduced. Increasing the drug concentration to improve effectiveness can lead to more systemic side effects. The following table evaluates five common factors of chemotherapy.

Chemotherapy Scorecard

Key Dimensions	Scores (out of 100)	The Reasons for the Scores.	Causes of Losing Points
Inhibition Rate	30	Systemic medication has a relatively low inhibition rate.	Drugs need to act over a long period, but maintaining concentration within the tumor is challenging.
Safety	10	Moderate safety.	Side effects are numerous, and increasing the inhibition rate tends to exacerbate them.
Drug Resistance	50	Resistance develops later.	Drug resistance is relatively common.
Sustainability	50	It can be used long-term.	However, as inhibition decreases, side effects increase.
Convenience	100	Very convenient.	
Average Score	48		

3. Radiation Therapy

Radiation therapy is a common medical technique used to treat cancer, employing high-energy radiation to kill cancer cells or inhibit their growth. This treatment can be delivered using external beam radiation machines or by placing radioactive substances directly near the tumor inside the body. It can be the primary treatment method or used in conjunction with chemotherapy, surgery, and other treatments to enhance effectiveness.

Before starting radiation therapy, doctors utilize advanced imaging technologies like CT scans, MRI, or PET scans to pinpoint the exact location and size of the tumor. This information helps radiation therapists accurately target the treatment area, minimizing damage to surrounding healthy tissue. The treatment plan is usually developed by a team of specialists, including radiation oncologists, medical physicists, and radiation therapists.

During radiation therapy, patients lie on a specially designed table and must remain still. The treatment machine moves around the patient, emitting radiation from multiple angles to precisely target the tumor. Each session typically lasts only a few minutes, though the entire treatment course may span several weeks, depending on the type and purpose of the treatment.

The goal of radiation therapy is to destroy as many cancer cells as possible while protecting the surrounding normal cells. To achieve this, treatments are often divided into multiple small doses, administered daily, allowing normal cells the chance to repair damage incurred during treatment. This approach of fractionating the dose helps improve the safety and effectiveness of the treatment.

Despite its high precision, radiation therapy can still affect surrounding normal tissues. During and after treatment, patients may experience side effects such as skin irritation, fatigue, and hair loss. The severity of these side effects varies from person to person and usually subsides after treatment ends.

With technological advancements, radiation therapy has become more precise and effective. Techniques like Intensity-Modulated Radiation Therapy (IMRT) allow doctors to adjust the intensity of the radiation beams, targeting the tumor more precisely while protecting more normal tissue. Another technique, Stereotactic Body Radiation Therapy (SBRT), enables precise targeting of small or well-defined tumors with higher doses in fewer sessions.

Over the past 50 years, significant progress has been made in radiation therapy technology, achieving a favorable balance between inhibition rates and side effects. However, the complexity and high cost of radiation therapy equipment remain drawbacks, making its use less convenient. The following table provides a detailed assessment of five key factors of radiation therapy.

Radiation Therapy Scorecard

Key Dimensions	Scores (out of 100)	The Reasons for the Scores.	Causes of Losing Points
Inhibition Rate	90	Physical methods are used to directly kill cancer cells.	Radiation therapy targets small areas and requires scanning.

Safety	60	New devices, such as proton therapy machines, offer high safety levels.	It can sometimes damage the immune system and cause inflammation.
Drug Resistance	70	Resistance to treatment is uncommon with these methods, allowing for long-term use.	Drug resistance is a possibility.
Sustainability	70	These devices are becoming increasingly common.	The complexity of the procedures has increased.
Convenience	50	Physical methods are used to directly kill cancer cells.	The equipment used is relatively large.
Average Score	68		

4. Targeted Therapy

Targeted drug therapy is a modern cancer treatment method that uses drugs to precisely attack specific molecular mechanisms in cancer cells, rather than affecting both healthy and cancerous cells as traditional chemotherapy does. This approach is based on a deep understanding of cancer biology, particularly the molecular and cellular processes involved in cancer cell growth and spread.

The development of targeted therapy drugs begins with the identification of biological markers unique to cancer cells. These biomarkers are specific proteins or genes that cancer cells rely on for survival and proliferation. By targeting these key biomarkers, targeted drugs can block the growth signals of cancer cells or alter their growth environment, thereby inhibiting tumor development.

A key advantage of targeted therapy is its selectivity, which allows the drugs to act more directly on cancer cells, reducing damage to normal cells. This typically results in fewer side effects compared to traditional chemotherapy, thus improving patients' quality of life.

A common form of targeted therapy involves the use of small molecule inhibitors. These drugs can enter cells and directly target specific proteins or signaling pathways. For example, some small molecule inhibitors block tyrosine kinases, enzymes that play a crucial role in the proliferation of many cancer cells.

Another type of targeted therapy involves monoclonal antibodies. These large molecule drugs are designed to recognize and bind to specific molecules on the surface of cancer cells, thereby triggering the immune system to attack the cancer cells or directly blocking the growth signals of the cancer cells. Monoclonal antibodies can also be engineered to carry toxins, radioactive substances, or other drugs, delivering these destructive agents directly to cancer cells without affecting surrounding healthy cells.

The effectiveness of targeted drug therapy depends on various factors, including the type of cancer, individual differences among patients, and the genetic characteristics of the tumor. Therefore, doctors may recommend molecular diagnostic testing before starting treatment to identify the specific genetic and molecular features of the tumor, enabling the selection of the most appropriate targeted drug.

Advances in cancer genomics and molecular biology are continually leading to the discovery and development of new targets and therapeutic drugs. These advancements not only increase the available treatment options but also enhance the precision and personalization of treatments.

In practice, targeted drug therapy can be used alone or in combination with other cancer treatments such as chemotherapy, radiation therapy, or immunotherapy. This multimodal treatment strategy aims to attack cancer from different angles to enhance therapeutic effects while minimizing the impact on the patient.

Although targeted drug therapy is highly effective in many cases, it also faces challenges such as the development of drug resistance. Cancer cells can mutate over time, developing resistance to targeted drugs, which necessitates ongoing adjustments and optimizations of treatment plans.

Targeted drugs generally show advantages over chemotherapy drugs in terms of short-term inhibition rates and safety, but due to significant drug resistance, their sustainability scores are lower. The following table provides a detailed assessment of five key factors of targeted therapy.

Targeted Therapy Scorecard

Key Dimensions	Scores (out of 100)	The Reasons for the Scores.	Causes of Losing Points
Inhibition Rate	50	They often outperform chemotherapy in inhibition rates.	Systemic medication, loss of concentration in the tumor

Safety	50	They are generally safer than chemotherapy.	Systemic medication, certain damage to normal cells
Drug Resistance	10	Drug resistance is quite common.	
Sustainability	50	These therapies allow for the flexibility to switch drugs as needed.	Tumor heterogeneity, the development of targeted drugs cannot keep up
Convenience	100	They offer significant convenience in treatment management.	
Average Score	52		

5. Tumor Ablation

Tumor ablation is a minimally invasive treatment for certain types of tumors, particularly in the liver, kidneys, and lungs. This technique destroys tumor cells by applying extreme temperatures directly, using various energy sources such as radiofrequency, microwaves, lasers, and cryotherapy. Each method has its unique approach and mechanism, but all aim to precisely eliminate tumor cells while preserving surrounding healthy tissue.

Radiofrequency ablation (RFA) uses radio waves to generate heat, destroying tumor cells by heating them to lethal temperatures. A thin needle-like electrode is inserted into the tumor, where it generates heat through electrical currents.

Microwave ablation (MWA) is similar to RFA but uses microwave energy to achieve higher temperatures and destroy tumor cells more quickly. It can treat larger tumors than RFA.

Laser ablation directs high-energy lasers at the tumor, converting light energy into heat to destroy the cells. A laser fiber is inserted through the skin into the tumor, allowing precise control over the laser's release to minimize damage to surrounding tissues.

Cryotherapy, also known as cryoablation, treats tumors by freezing the cells with extremely low temperatures. Liquid nitrogen or argon gas is delivered to the tumor through a thin probe, rapidly lowering the temperature and forming ice crystals that disrupt cell structures, leading to cell death.

Tumor ablation is usually performed under local anesthesia or mild sedation, depending on the ablation method and the size of the treatment area. During the procedure, imaging techniques like ultrasound, CT scans, or MRI may be used to guide and monitor the probe's position, ensuring energy is accurately delivered to the tumor.

Due to its minimally invasive nature, tumor ablation often results in shorter recovery times and lower risks of postoperative pain and complications compared to traditional open surgery. This makes it a viable option for patients who may not be suitable for conventional surgery.

Tumor ablation is suitable for patients with smaller, well-defined tumors and is particularly beneficial for those who cannot undergo traditional surgery due to age or other health issues. It can also serve as a supplementary treatment for patients whose tumors have not been completely removed or are at risk of recurrence.

Photodynamic therapy (PDT) is another form of tumor ablation that combines a photosensitizing agent with a specific wavelength of light. This treatment involves administering a photosensitizer to the patient, which accumulates in the tumor cells. After a period, the treated area is exposed to light of a specific wavelength. The light's energy, absorbed by the photosensitizer, generates reactive oxygen species or free radicals that destroy the tumor cells.

PDT's advantage lies in its high selectivity, primarily targeting tumor cells that have accumulated the photosensitizer, causing minimal damage to surrounding healthy tissue. Side effects are generally mild, mainly photosensitivity reactions where the patient's skin and eyes may become more sensitive to light for some time after treatment.

PDT is primarily used for treating superficial tumors, such as skin cancer and certain types of head and neck cancers. It can also be used as an adjunct treatment for some internal tumors, for example, by guiding light to specific internal sites through an endoscope. In some cases, PDT is also used to treat non-cancerous conditions like macular degeneration.

The effectiveness of PDT depends on several factors, including the type of photosensitizer, the wavelength of light, the duration of exposure, and the type and location of the tumor. As new photosensitizers and more precise light sources are developed, the scope and expected outcomes of PDT are likely to improve further.

Tumor ablation is technically similar to radiation therapy but uses smaller, more portable, and sustainable equipment, typically with fewer side effects than radiation therapy. The following table provides a detailed assessment of five key factors of tumor ablation.

Tumor Ablation Scorecard

Key Dimensions	Scores (out of 100)	The Reasons for the Scores.	Causes of Losing Points
Inhibition Rate	90	Physical methods effectively eliminate cancer cells.	Physical methods are limited by tumor size and shape.
Safety	80	They are safer than radiation therapy.	Some techniques may damage normal tissue.
Drug Resistance	100	There is no risk of drug resistance.	Treatment becomes challenging when there are multiple tumors.
Sustainability	70	These methods can be used repeatedly.	When tumors are numerous or large, the procedure becomes more complex.
Convenience	60	They are generally more convenient.	Physical methods are limited by tumor size and shape.
Average Score	78		

6. Immunotherapy

Cancer immunotherapy is a treatment that harnesses the power of the human immune system to recognize and attack cancer cells. This therapy builds on the immune system's natural function to protect the body from diseases. Normally, the immune system can identify and eliminate abnormal cells, including cancer cells. However, cancer cells often find ways to evade immune surveillance. The goal of cancer immunotherapy is to enhance the immune system's natural functions to help it more effectively identify and attack cancer cells.

One common form of cancer immunotherapy is immune checkpoint inhibitors. Immune checkpoints are mechanisms on the immune system that prevent immune cells from attacking normal cells. Cancer cells can exploit these checkpoints to protect themselves from immune attacks. Immune checkpoint inhibitors work by blocking these checkpoints, removing the cancer cells' "invisibility cloak" and allowing the immune system to detect and destroy them. For example, PD-1 and CTLA-4 are two immune checkpoints commonly exploited by cancer cells, and inhibitors targeting these can effectively activate the immune system against cancer.

Another strategy is cell therapy, such as CAR-T cell therapy. This involves extracting T cells (a type of immune cell) from the patient's body, genetically modifying them in the laboratory to better recognize cancer cells, and then reintroducing these modified cells—known as Chimeric Antigen Receptor T cells (CAR-T)—back into the patient to attack cancer cells. This treatment has shown high efficacy in certain types of blood cancer.

Cancer vaccines are another form of immunotherapy designed to stimulate the immune system's response to specific cancers. These vaccines typically contain specific antigens from cancer cells, which can activate the immune system to recognize and attack cells containing these antigens. Cancer vaccines can be preventative, aimed at preventing cancer from developing, or therapeutic, intended to treat existing cancer.

Immunomodulators are drugs that adjust the activity of the immune system, enhancing or modulating the immune response through various mechanisms. For example, some immunomodulators can enhance the ability of immune cells to attack cancer cells or alter the immune environment to be more conducive to immune system activity.

The research and application of cancer immunotherapy is a rapidly evolving field. As our understanding of the immune system and cancer biology deepens, new treatment methods continue to be developed. These therapies offer a different approach from traditional surgery, radiation, and chemotherapy, providing hope for some hard-to-treat cancers.

Despite the success of cancer immunotherapy in many cases, it also faces challenges. Not all patients respond to this treatment, and sometimes immunotherapy can trigger severe immune-related side effects. Therefore, scientists and doctors are striving to better understand which patients are most likely to benefit from immunotherapy and how to manage potential side effects during treatment. Additionally, researchers are exploring how to combine immunotherapy with other forms of cancer treatment to enhance treatment outcomes.

The development of immunotherapy still focuses on targeting specific points, thus facing similar side effects and resistance issues as targeted drugs. However, its advantage lies in its mechanism, which aligns with the long-term goals of cancer treatment: by activating the immune system and combining it with other therapies, a comprehensive effect can be achieved. The following table provides a detailed assessment of five key factors of immunotherapy.

Immunotherapy Scorecard

Key Dimensions	Scores (out of 100)	The Reasons for the Scores.	Causes of Losing Points
Inhibition Rate	70	This method effectively kills tumors using the immune system.	Activating the immune system has limitations and targets tumors selectively.
Safety	70	It is safer than targeted drugs.	It can trigger autoimmune diseases easily.
Drug Resistance	40	However, resistance can develop.	The resistance mechanism is similar to targeted drugs.
Sustainability	60	It can be used continuously with other therapies.	However, sustainability is compromised due to resistance.
Convenience	90	Most approved therapies are quite convenient.	Some specific immunotherapies are quite complex.
Average Score	66		

7. Comprehensive Comparison

Using the same approach, we can apply the five-factor analysis framework to any cancer treatment. Here, we compared six common cancer treatment methods. According to the scoring results, tumor ablation emerged as the most effective, suggesting it should be the preferred method if patient-specific conditions are not considered. In contrast, chemotherapy received the lowest overall score, indicating that patients might consider avoiding it. However, the potential of combination therapies should not be overlooked. For example, combining tumor ablation with chemotherapy, using methods like intra-tumor injections of chemotherapy drugs similar to those used at the "Baofa" Hospital in China, might be considered off-label in the current medical system but could offer superior treatment outcomes.

Cancer Treatments Comprehensive Scorecard

Key Dimensions	Surgical	Chemotherapy	Radiation Therapy	Targeted Therapy	Tumor Ablation	Immunotherapy
Inhibition Rate	100	30	90	50	90	70
Safety	50	10	60	50	80	70
Drug Resistance	100	50	70	10	100	40
Sustainability	10	50	70	50	70	60

Cancer Treatments Comprehensive Scorecard

Convenience	30	100	50	100	60	90
Average Score	58	48	68	52	78	66

In reality, cancer patients often undergo various treatment methods, making combination therapy a recommended approach. This method is similar to evaluating single therapies, and our analysis framework is equally applicable to assessing combination therapies composed of multiple treatments. While this adds complexity to the evaluation process, it holds significant value for patients.

Through comprehensive assessment tables, we can propose and evaluate various potential combination therapies, selecting the optimal approach based on scores, even if the therapy does not currently exist. For instance, combining surgery with immunotherapy may be more effective than combining tumor ablation with immunotherapy. By refining specific therapies within a reasonable framework, such as not completely excising tumors during surgery but primarily disrupting tumor vasculature and directly injecting immunotherapy drugs into the tumor, we may not only reduce surgical complexity but also release antigens and stimulate immune responses in the tumor microenvironment, potentially achieving better treatment outcomes.

Furthermore, we can further adjust existing combination therapies using first principles, such as exploring the possibility of delivering immunotherapy drugs directly during tumor ablation, an adjustment to the combination of tumor ablation and immunotherapy, similar to the treatment approaches focused on by the Williams Cancer Institute in the United States.

Therefore, if cancer patients understand the application of first principles in cancer treatment, they can evaluate both single therapies and combination therapies through the same process. They can not only assess these therapies but also make reasonable adjustments within the existing healthcare system. This deepens patients' understanding of their cancer, alleviates psychological burdens, and contributes to effective cancer treatment and the goal of achieving long-term high-quality life.

PART FOUR: THE FUTURE DIRECTION OF CANCER TREATMENT

First Principles Thinking is a problem-solving approach that involves breaking down a problem into its most fundamental principles or basic truths, and then constructing solutions from the ground up. At SpaceX, First Principles Thinking is extensively applied in the design and development of rockets and spacecraft to ensure innovative and efficient solutions.

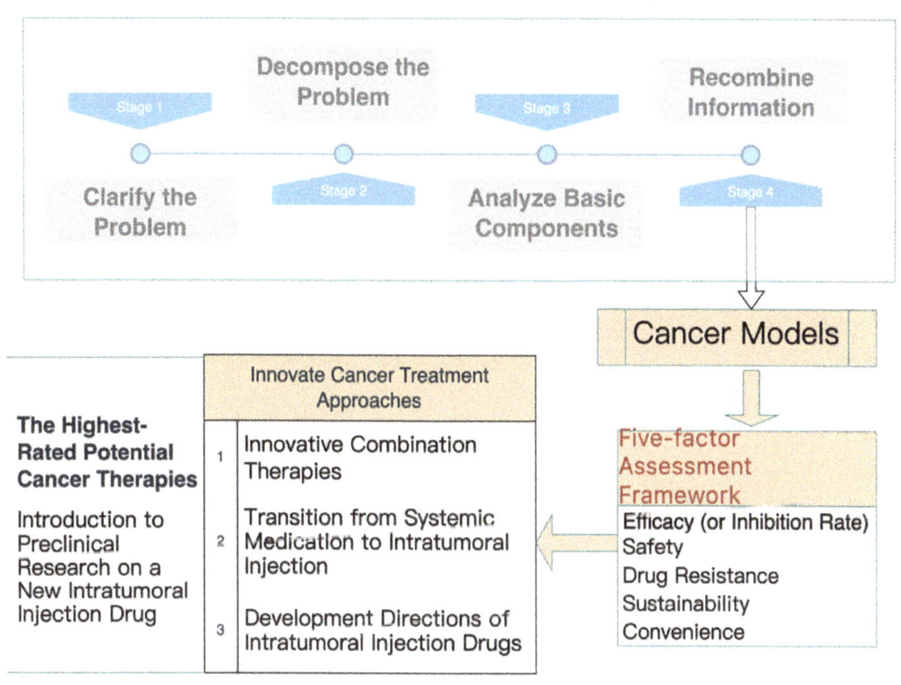

Decompose the Problem
Recombine Information
Stage 1
Stage 3
Clarify the Problem
Stage 2
Analyze Basic Components
Stage 4
Cancer Models
Innovate Cancer Treatment Approaches
The Highest-Rated Potential Cancer Therapies
Introduction to Preclinical Research on a New Intratumoral Injection Drug
1 Innovative Combination Therapies
2 Transition from Systemic Medication to Intratumoral Injection
3 Development Directions of Intratumoral Injection Drugs
Five-factor Assessment Framework
Efficacy (or Inhibition Rate)
Safety
Drug Resistance
Sustainability
Convenience

First principles are a method of problem-solving that involves breaking down existing assumptions to the most fundamental truths or facts. This approach requires us to discard traditional assumptions and empirical rules, starting from the most basic facts and logic to rebuild our understanding of the problem and its solutions.

By applying first principles, both individuals and organizations can gain deeper insights into the essence of problems, avoiding reliance on traditional methods, and potentially discovering more effective and innovative solutions. This method encourages deep thinking and innovation, helping to break conventions and explore new possibilities.

In earlier chapters, we redesigned the analysis model and evaluation framework for cancer treatment using first principles. Although the discussed cancer therapies are still traditional, approved, and listed in the NCCN guidelines, our innovation lies not only in the specific cancer therapies but also in the approach to choosing cancer treatments.

While implementing innovative cancer therapies is nearly impossible for the average patient within the current healthcare system, we can still use our learned thinking approach to envision better cancer treatment options that may emerge in the future.

9.1 Innovative Combination Therapies

In the previous chapter, we evaluated six common cancer therapies using a five-factor framework derived from first principles. We found that combining these therapies could result in higher overall scores, forming better treatment options. In this chapter, we will continue to apply first principles, combine these six cancer therapies, explore new treatment combinations, and evaluate them using the same five-factor framework.

Firstly, we will display these six cancer therapy combinations on a two-dimensional graph, using inhibition rate and immune enhancement (and their associated side effects) to demonstrate their effectiveness in a single cancer treatment. In this graph, we use PDT to represent tumor ablation and CD to represent innovative combination therapies.

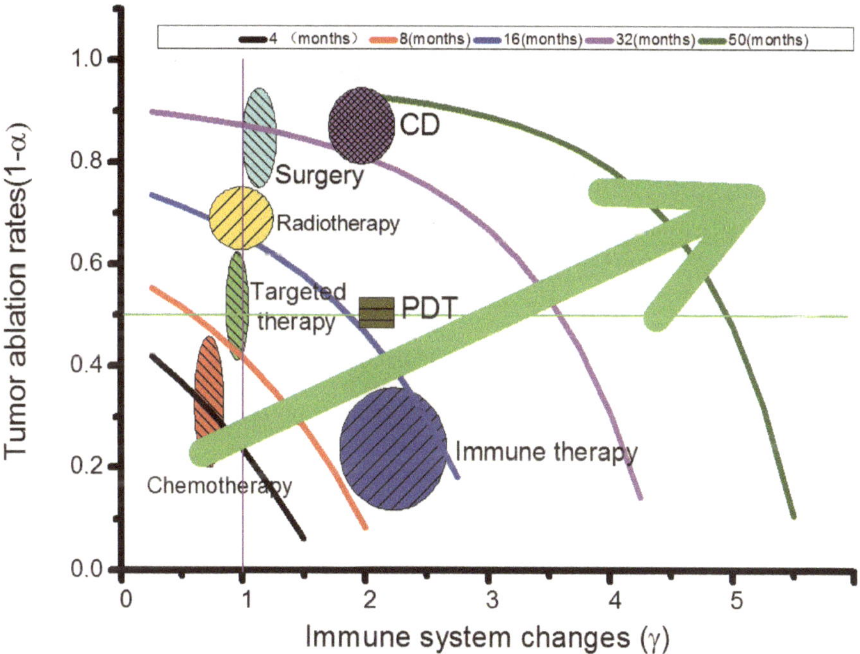

The combined effect of tumor ablation rates and additional immune enhancement on extending survival. The approach to cancer treatment always involves choosing between directly eliminating cancer cells or relying on immune cells to clear cancer cells. Ideally, enhancing both methods is the most effective treatment approach. Existing treatment plans generate different combinations of these two methods, each with varying effects

(survival extension). Targeted therapy and surgery only affect ablation rates; chemotherapy also impacts ablation rates but harms immune capabilities; radiation therapy affects ablation rates and has a slight immune enhancement effect; immunotherapy primarily boosts immune capabilities, relying on the immune system to suppress tumors again; PDT can directly ablate tumors and trigger an anti-tumor immune response, but its complex procedure and limited depth of tumor penetration result in lower ablation rates; CD (an ideal combination therapy) can directly ablate tumors, potentially trigger an immune response, and is easy to use. The combination approach to tumor treatment should aim to expand the combined effect towards the top right corner: increasing direct ablation rates and enhancing anti-tumor immune capabilities.

The horizontal axis in the graph represents immune enhancement, while the vertical axis represents cancer suppression rate (or ablation rate). The curves concaving towards the origin in the coordinate system represent isopleths of cancer therapy prolonging survival, meaning that on any curve, the same survival extension is indicated.

When designing tumor treatment combinations, our goal is to drive treatment effects towards the top right corner, simultaneously increasing direct ablation rates and enhancing anti-tumor immune capabilities. This combination strategy aims to achieve better treatment outcomes by integrating the advantages of multiple treatment methods.

Since a two-dimensional graph can only display two factors, we will gradually introduce the other three factors in the upcoming analysis. The following table will be used to analyze various possible cancer therapy combinations.

COMBINATION THERAPIES

	Surgical	Chemotherapy	Radiation Therapy	Targeted Therapy	Tumor Ablation	Immunotherapy
Surgical		6				3
Chemotherapy	6			4		2
Radiation Therapy				2		1
Targeted Therapy		4	2			
Tumor Ablation						5
Immunotherapy	3	2	1		5	

When analyzing the pairwise combinations of cancer treatment methods, we can look for those that perform weakly in certain key dimensions but strongly in others to achieve complementary advantages. Here are several complementary combinations derived from the data analysis of the scoring table of the six cancer therapies from the previous chapter:

(1) Radiation Therapy + Immunotherapy

- Radiation therapy provides high suppression rates and good sustainability but has moderate convenience.
- Immunotherapy enhances convenience and sustainability, boosting patients' immune responses. This combination is quite common in clinical practice as radiation therapy can promote antigen release, significantly enhancing immune capabilities when combined with immunotherapy.

(2) Chemotherapy + Immunotherapy

- Chemotherapy is highly convenient but may pose lower safety and drug resistance issues.
- Immunotherapy can improve safety and drug resistance while enhancing long-term treatment outcomes. This combination is frequently seen in clinical practice, with the complementary advantages of two different therapies.

(3) Surgery + Immunotherapy

- Surgery offers the highest suppression rates but lower sustainability and convenience.
- Immunotherapy helps enhance the long-term effects and convenience of surgery. This combination is less common, but adjustments can be made, such as not completely removing the tumor during surgery but primarily disrupting the tumor's blood vessels and delivering immune drugs directly into the tumor. This approach may reduce the complexity of surgery, release antigens, and trigger an immune response in the tumor microenvironment, potentially leading to better treatment outcomes.

(4) Chemotherapy + Targeted Therapy

- Although chemotherapy is highly convenient, it has lower safety and drug resistance.

- Targeted therapy improves drug resistance and safety while increasing suppression rates. This combination is also quite common, especially in delaying the emergence of drug resistance to targeted therapy in the future. Using chemotherapy appropriately can inhibit resistant cancer cells because chemotherapy resistance is weaker than targeted drug resistance.

(5) Tumor Ablation + Immunotherapy

- Tumor ablation scores high in safety and drug resistance but may require support in suppression rates and sustainability.
- Immunotherapy provides sustained treatment effects, enhancing immune surveillance after tumor ablation. This combination is already present in clinical practice, especially in clinical trials with immunotherapy drugs, where tumor ablation is its best combination. The reason lies in tumor ablation's ability to release antigens, enhancing the effectiveness of immunotherapy.

(6) Chemotherapy + Surgery

- Chemotherapy offers convenience and initial tumor control.
- Surgery can precisely remove residual tumors, and their combination can improve overall treatment success rates. This combination is also common in clinical practice, especially when dealing with larger tumors. Using chemotherapy drugs to shrink the tumor appropriately before surgery can facilitate tumor removal.

9.2 Transition from Systemic Medication to Intratumoral Injection

In cancer treatment, drug therapy plays a crucial role due to the development of new medications targeting various molecular mechanisms. With potentially hundreds of gene mutations present in cancer tissues, theoretically, a new drug could be developed for each target, leading to the possibility of thousands of new drugs. However, most cancer drugs are administered orally or through intravenous injection, resulting in systemic distribution of the medication and low drug concentrations at the tumor site, along with inevitable systemic side effects.

Traditionally, systemic drug use is essential during the research and development process to explore the causes of tumors, which are often related to the overall bodily systems, such as gene mutations, DNA replication errors, and metabolic issues. While breaking away from this tradition is challenging, applying first principles allows us to explore new approaches.

To enhance the inhibitory effects of drugs and reduce side effects, directly delivering medications to tumor tissues is a straightforward solution. Although this method faces challenges regarding the short retention time of drugs in tumors, its effectiveness surpasses systemic drug administration. Some medical institutions have started to explore innovative treatments, such as intratumoral chemotherapy at China's Baofa Hospital and intratumoral immunotherapy at the Williams Cancer

Institute in the United States. These pioneers not only utilize intratumoral injections but also combine them with tumor ablation to treat patients collectively.

One significant challenge of intratumoral injections is the brief drug retention time within tumors. Future research directions may involve developing new drug materials to prolong drug retention in tumors. With advancing technology, intratumoral injection methods will likely simplify over time, potentially becoming a significant trend in future cancer treatment. This approach could also serve as a crucial pathway for new drug development and earn a place in future NCCN guidelines.

9.3 Development Directions of Intratumoral Injection Drugs

In the earlier part, we talked about the emerging trend where current cancer medications may transition towards intratumoral injection. Although localized delivery can improve inhibition rates and minimize adverse effects, conventional drugs encounter challenges in remaining within tumors long enough to maintain tumor suppression. Moreover, intratumoral injection falls short in tackling drug resistance and sustainability concerns. This approach prioritizes increased inhibition rates and reduced side effects over convenience.

Innovative approaches are required to tackle drug resistance, particularly concerning cancer treatment. By once again applying first principles, we emphasize the deconstruction of fundamental components at the cellular level when applied to cancer therapy, which is crucial in overcoming reductionist influences in modern medical research.

Modern medical research heavily influenced by reductionism often delves into exploring biology at a more intricate level, reaching the molecular level when searching for root causes. New drug research must possess clear molecular mechanisms, especially concerning cancer, where gene mutations become the target of the majority of new drugs. In this model, treatment targets also reside at the molecular level. However, complex issues like drug resistance often present numerous unpredictable challenges at the systemic level. Due to the heterogeneity of cancer tissues, a tumor may harbor hundreds of different mutations, with a targeted drug typically only inhibiting one type of mutated cancer cell. Following this inhibition, other drug-resistant cancer cells may proliferate faster, sometimes even surpassing the speed of proliferation without targeted drug treatment.

Even immunotherapies, developed from the perspective of targeting immune cells, face drug resistance issues. For instance, PD-1 drugs, as immune checkpoint inhibitors, enhance the immune system's ability to attack cancer cells by blocking the PD-1 and its ligand binding, yet drug resistance remains a concern. The emergence of drug resistance primarily stems from changes in the tumor microenvironment, tumor heterogeneity, and immune escape mechanisms. These factors indicate that drug development based on subcellular levels inevitably encounters drug resistance issues.

Therefore, when analyzing cancer treatment using first principles, a focus on the cellular level is crucial. Next, let's examine the major issues of the intratumoral drug injection model:

(1) Selective Cancer Cell Killing: Even chemotherapy drugs may exhibit some selectivity, implying they may not effectively target all types of cancer cells. (2) Slow Killing Action: Compared to physical methods like tumor ablation, drug-induced cancer cell killing occurs more slowly, with physical methods capable of killing most cancer cells within minutes. (3) Activation of Immune Response: The way drugs kill cancer cells may not efficiently generate antigens like tumor ablation does to activate an anti-tumor immune response. (4) Impact on Tumor Vasculature: Cancer cells, as originally normal cells, require more energy, primarily supplied through the tumor tissue's blood vessels. Current intratumoral injection drugs seem incapable of destroying tumor blood vessels.

These issues highlight the limitations of the intratumoral injection drug model in practical application, suggesting the need for more innovative treatment strategies to overcome these challenges.

For the aforementioned four issues, the following solutions can be proposed: Firstly, to address the first point, developing a non-selective drug that can kill cancer cells indiscriminately (currently approved drugs lack this property); secondly, for the second point, selecting drugs capable of instantly killing cancer cells; thirdly, for the third point, developing drugs that can utilize the immune system to kill cancer cells, thereby releasing antigens while killing cancer cells; finally, for the fourth point, seeking substances that can rapidly destroy tumor blood vessels.

For the average cancer patient, finding such substances and solving the above four issues is nearly impossible. However, as the author of this book, I have discovered such a substance and completed preclinical research. In the following sections, I will provide a detailed introduction to this preclinical research. Additionally, in the extended portion of this book, I will attach the complete paper for professionals to review.

9.4 Introduction to Preclinical Research on a New Intratumoral Injection Drug[4]

I. Research Summary

Our team is currently exploring the potential use of chlorine dioxide in cancer treatment. Chlorine dioxide, with properties similar to reactive oxygen species (ROS), has demonstrated the ability to destroy cancer cells and support tissue repair. We have found that chlorine dioxide can be safely utilized as a therapeutic agent in humans. Our research involves delivering chlorine dioxide directly into tumors as an innovative approach to cancer treatment. By targeting tumors specifically, chlorine dioxide can effectively kill cancer cells without fostering drug resistance. Moreover, chlorine dioxide has shown the capacity to stimulate an immune response against cancer, enhancing its therapeutic impact. Our objective is to prolong patients' lives and transform cancer into a manageable chronic

---

[4] Regarding the complete preclinical research report on this intratumoral injection drug, we offer it in the Further Reading section for readers with expertise to review.

condition by injecting chlorine dioxide directly into tumors. This groundbreaking treatment leverages chlorine dioxide's ROS-mimicking properties to eradicate cancer cells and encourage tissue regeneration. Through harnessing chlorine dioxide's unique characteristics, we offer a novel route to enhance patient outcomes in cancer treatment. Ongoing studies are essential to optimize the delivery methods and dosage of chlorine dioxide, as well as explore its synergistic effects with other treatments. As research progresses, direct tumor injection of chlorine dioxide emerges as a promising and exciting approach to effective cancer therapy.

II. Introduction to the Research

Certain natural compounds or drugs targeting Superoxide dismutase (SOD) possess the remarkable ability to selectively eliminate cancer cells by increasing reactive oxygen species (ROS) production or accumulation. Neutrophils within the body can also generate ROS, aiding in cancer cell destruction. Some drugs are specifically designed to elevate ROS levels within cancer cells, leading to sustained disease suppression. For example, the combination of metformin, which boosts ROS levels, and apigenin, which enhances this effect, demonstrates potent anticancer action while sparing healthy cells. Photodynamic therapy (PDT) is another method utilizing light to activate a photosensitizer drug, producing singlet oxygen (1O2) in the body. This sudden oxygen surge induces toxicity in tumor cells, resulting in cell death through apoptosis or necrosis. PDT not only targets and eliminates tumors directly but also triggers dendritic cells to release cell death-associated molecular patterns (DAMPs), initiating an immune response that targets antigens and promotes an anti-tumor immune reaction.

Expanding on this concept, our hypothesis suggests that the external application of ROS or similar compounds could effectively eradicate tumors and, akin to PDT, trigger an antitumor immune response. In this context, we have selected chlorine dioxide as a ROS-mimicking oxidant to assess its potential in cancer treatment. Chlorine dioxide, represented by its chemical formula ClO_2, is a potent oxidizing agent with disinfectant properties. Its applications span various fields, including water purification, food sanitation, medical sterilization, and environmental decontamination. Chlorine dioxide efficiently breaks down the cell membranes and DNA of bacteria, viruses, and other microbes, effectively eliminating pathogens and impurities. Notably, at a low concentration of 0.25 mg/L, chlorine dioxide can eradicate 99% of E. coli (15,000 cells/mL) within just 15 seconds. Additionally, research has shown that chlorine dioxide and hydrogen peroxide have similar effectiveness in inducing cell death in human gingival fibroblasts.

ROS are generated during cellular respiration for ATP synthesis. However, the extensive ROS production in the body and the limited capacity to rapidly eliminate a significant number of cells, especially within tumor tissues, pose significant challenges. These challenges are predominantly attributed to tumor hypoxia, characterized by low oxygen levels in the tumor environment. To set a new standard for cancer treatment, it is vital to elevate chlorine dioxide concentrations to a level where it can effectively eradicate large tumor masses, surpassing the body's natural ROS production. Furthermore, due to chlorine dioxide's short lifespan as an oxidizing agent in body tissues and the necessity to minimize systemic side effects, we have opted for intratumoral administration of chlorine dioxide as the most effective method to achieve our objective.

III. Research Results and Discussion

This study investigated the effects of chlorine dioxide on tumors and tissues using mice as subjects, yielding intriguing findings. Chlorine dioxide displayed toxicity towards both cancer and normal cells without specific targeting. Upon injection beneath the mice's skin, it caused significant skin damage. However, within approximately 20 days, the damaged tissue fully healed, returning to its normal state and regrowing hair. This indicates that while chlorine dioxide may harm tissues, the body possesses the ability to self-repair.

To assess wound healing, cuts were made on the mice's tails. Mice treated with chlorine dioxide or hydrogen peroxide experienced accelerated wound closure compared to those treated with a saline solution alone, with wounds healing approximately 6 days earlier. Chlorine dioxide seemed to assist in the removal of dead tissue debris near the wounds, potentially contributing to the healing process.

Moreover, direct injection of chlorine dioxide into tumors in mice led to a significant inhibition of tumor growth. The tumors reduced in size, displaying signs of dead tissue within them. Additionally, chlorine dioxide administration notably reduced cancer spread to the lungs.

Researchers proposed two mechanisms by which chlorine dioxide operates. Firstly, it induces cancer cell death through apoptosis (programmed cell death) and necrosis (cell death due to injury or disease). Secondly, it triggers an immune response against cancer, potentially enhancing its therapeutic effects.

IV. Research Summary

Our study has revealed the versatile potential of chlorine dioxide as a promising cancer therapy. Chlorine dioxide, akin to reactive oxygen species (ROS), exhibits regenerative properties that can enhance tissue repair. This quality positions it as a valuable candidate for improving wound healing within cancer treatment, considering tumors as challenging wounds to heal. By harnessing chlorine dioxide's regenerative abilities, we aim to enhance patient recovery throughout cancer therapy.

Chlorine dioxide therapy presents numerous advantages over conventional cancer treatments. It not only mitigates disease-related complications and risks but also offers a safer and more efficient alternative. Our proposed strategy of directly administering chlorine dioxide to the tumor site enables precise tumor eradication without encountering resistance, while also bolstering the body's anti-cancer immune response. This targeted method preserves healthy tissue and leverages chlorine dioxide's healing potential post-tumor removal, with the goal of optimizing treatment outcomes.

The landscape of oncology is undergoing a significant shift, propelled by immune checkpoint inhibitors. Ongoing clinical trials explore innovative approaches like intratumoral delivery and tumor-specific compounds, showing promise in enhancing drug concentration locally and amplifying the efficacy of immunotherapies. As novel technologies emerge, intratumoral chlorine dioxide administration emerges as a practical, effective, and patient-centric approach to cancer treatment. This technique holds the promise of extending patient lifespans and easing the treatment burden, transforming cancer management into a more chronic illness-oriented paradigm.

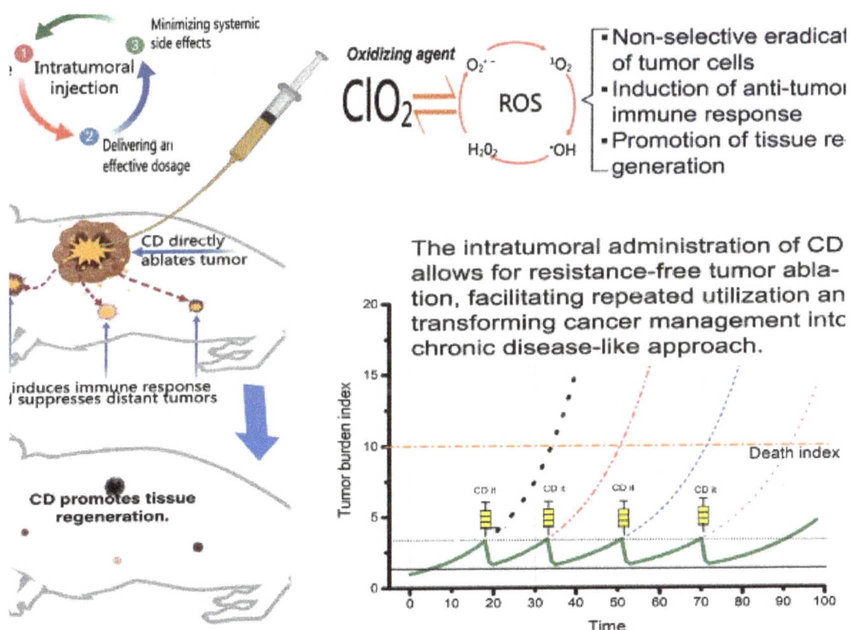

To fully capitalize on the potential of chlorine dioxide in cancer treatment, ongoing research is essential. It is necessary to refine the administration protocols, determine the optimal dosages, assess its compatibility with other treatments, and develop a thorough understanding of its impacts on tumor tissues in terms of both regeneration and destruction. Additionally, understanding its ability to provoke a systemic anti-cancer immune response is crucial. Recent studies have revealed a novel action of chlorine dioxide; when injected into tumors, it can destroy the tumor's blood vessels, cutting off its energy supply, which enhances its original inhibitory rate and safety.

Aligned with the preceding discussion, evaluating an ideal cancer treatment method involves considering five key dimensions: convenience, safety, inhibition rate, drug resistance, and treatment sustainability. According to the data in the provided table, intratumoral injection of chlorine dioxide excels in all these aspects, establishing it as an optimal method for cancer treatment.

Scoring chart for chlorine dioxide in cancer treatment

Key dimensions	Scores (out of 100)	The Reasons for the Scores.	Causes of Losing Points
Convenience	50	With the advancement of puncture techniques, intra-tumor injection is becoming increasingly easier.	It is less convenient than oral and intravenous injection.

Safety	95	The greatest advantage of intra-tumor injection is the absence of systemic side effects.	Inevitably, it causes some damage to normal tissues.
Inhibition Rate	100	Multiple pathways to inhibit injected tumors.	The inhibitory rate for tumors not injected remains relatively low.
Drug Resistance	100	Kills cancer cells without selection, eliminating drug resistance.	
Sustainability	95	It can be used repeatedly for long-term sustainability.	The convenience of intratumoral injection is relatively low.
Average Score	88		

When comparing intratumoral injection of chlorine dioxide cancer therapy with other conventional treatments, especially based on our five-factor evaluation framework, intratumoral injection of chlorine dioxide cancer treatment excels in aspects beyond convenience. In this scenario, the comprehensive score of intratumoral injection of chlorine dioxide significantly surpasses traditional cancer treatment methods. Considering the continuous improvement in the convenience of intratumoral injection with technological advancements, the cancer treatment with intratumoral injection of chlorine dioxide will have a competitive edge over traditional methods. It can be inferred that intratumoral injection of chlorine dioxide cancer treatment may transform cancer into a chronic disease, with most patients unlikely to succumb to cancer. This treatment does not rely on complex technologies but rather represents a breakthrough in treatment mindset. When cancer evolves into a chronic disease, patients will essentially not endure the current pressures, making overtreatment in cancer care highly improbable.

PART FIVE: FURTHER READING

This section is intended for readers with expertise. It includes the construction process of a mathematical model for life sciences, a preclinical study report currently under submission, and the development process of a cancer mathematical model based on the aforementioned work.

10. MATHEMATICAL MODEL OF LIFE

According to Schrödinger's description, life is a process that resists the entropy increase of the second law of thermodynamics. Life maintains its entropy by extracting energy, preventing it from increasing or decreasing (negative entropy). Entropy is defined as:

$$dS = \frac{dQ}{T}$$

Negative entropy is a broad concept that cannot fully describe the entire process of life. Assuming that an organism is composed entirely of cells, entropy characterizes the level of order in the organism. The increase in entropy signifies the transition of the organism from an ordered structure to a disordered one, which can be reflected by the overall order of the cells. When dysfunctional cells, such as aging cells or cancer cells, disrupt the order of the organism, the level of order decreases. Let's further assume that these poorly performing cells, or cells that lead to the loss of order in the organism, are collectively referred to as aging cells (including various dysfunctional and malignantly proliferating cells, with their main side effects being spatial occupation and disorder). The proportion of aging cells to the total cells is used to indicate the degree of disorder in the organism. This proportion is a straightforward way to reflect entropy increase because of its intuitive nature.

10.1 Model Establishment

The total number of cells in the human body is approximately 50×10^{12}. When the proportion of dysfunctional aging cells to the total cells reaches a certain level, around 1/3 in this case, the functions of various systems in the body will fail, leading to death. It is assumed that the total number of cells in the human body increases following a logistic model after birth.

$$\frac{dN}{dt} = rN(1 - \frac{N}{K})$$

Around the age of 20, the human body reaches its maximum mass, and the number of normal cells remains relatively constant until death. Therefore, with r=0.4 and $K=50\times10^{12}$, it is easy to derive the growth curve of human body cells (Fig.1).

After birth, due to environmental or internal system influences, body cells undergo various losses. Once these losses reach a certain level, cells start to age. Under the action of the immune system, these aging cells are cleared, but this clearance is not complete. We directly characterize the performance of the immune system in clearing aging cells by using the characteristics of the immune system in clearing cancer cells, which means that the immune system's clearance ability gradually decreases over time (the theory of immune editing, where cancer cells ultimately escape the immune system due to the decreasing clearance ability over time). This is a crucial variable as it reflects how aging in the human body affects the immune system and how artificially altering the immune system can have long-term effects on the clearance ability of aging cells. Human body cells also have a lifespan; they do not suddenly become aging cells at a fixed point in time but gradually accumulate losses until they reach a certain threshold to become aging cells. Moreover, these losses are likely to affect all cells rather than just a subset. Therefore, as time progresses, the number of aging cells increases at an accelerating rate. Assuming that the immune system's clearance ability is represented by a function: $\rho(t, \beta)$, where ρ represents the proportion of aging cells cleared by the immune system. We define the initial value of this function as β, which then decreases over time t.

At a certain point in time, the increase in the number of aging cells is:

$$\frac{dV}{dt} = K_1 V (1 - \rho(t, \beta)),$$

K_1 reflects the accumulation of losses in the body. We directly provide an approximate integral expression:

$$V(t) = e^{K_1 t} - \beta \frac{e^{K_1 t} e^{-K_2 t}}{1 + \beta e^{-K_2 t}}$$

K_1 reflects the immune system's decreasing coefficient according to a certain pattern. When aging cells account for 1/3 of all cells, the human body dies. This is the intersection point of the aging cell curve and the death line. Because organisms (such as humans) accumulate damage throughout their lives, and as individuals age, the immune system's ability to clear aging cells weakens. Therefore, the older a person gets, the faster the growth rate of aging cells that are not cleared, showing that the proportion of aging cells in the latter half of life grows exponentially.

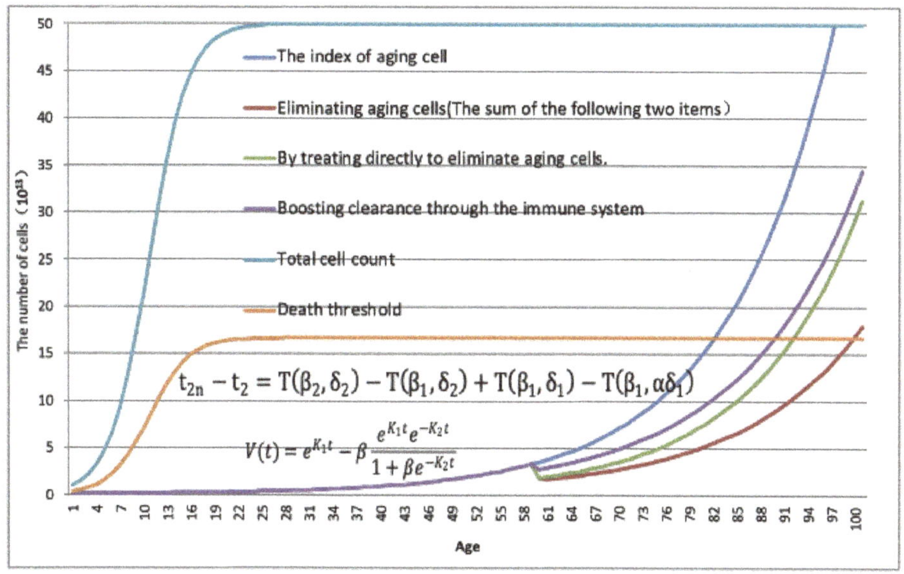

$$t_{2n} - t_2 = T(\beta_2, \delta_2) - T(\beta_1, \delta_2) + T(\beta_1, \delta_1) - T(\beta_1, \alpha\delta_1)$$

$$V(t) = e^{K_1 t} - \beta \frac{e^{K_1 t} e^{-K_2 t}}{1 + \beta e^{-K_2 t}}$$

Fig.1

10.2　Model Validation

1.Life Expectancy and Volume

A good theoretical model should accurately reflect reality or experimental results and, more importantly, have predictive capabilities. We can use several basic real-world principles to assess the correctness of our model. There is a rule in the animal kingdom: the heavier (or larger in volume) an adult animal is, the longer its maximum lifespan. The volume of adult animals can explain 63% of their maximum lifespan (1). As shown in the graph below, animal volume and lifespan are positively correlated.

155

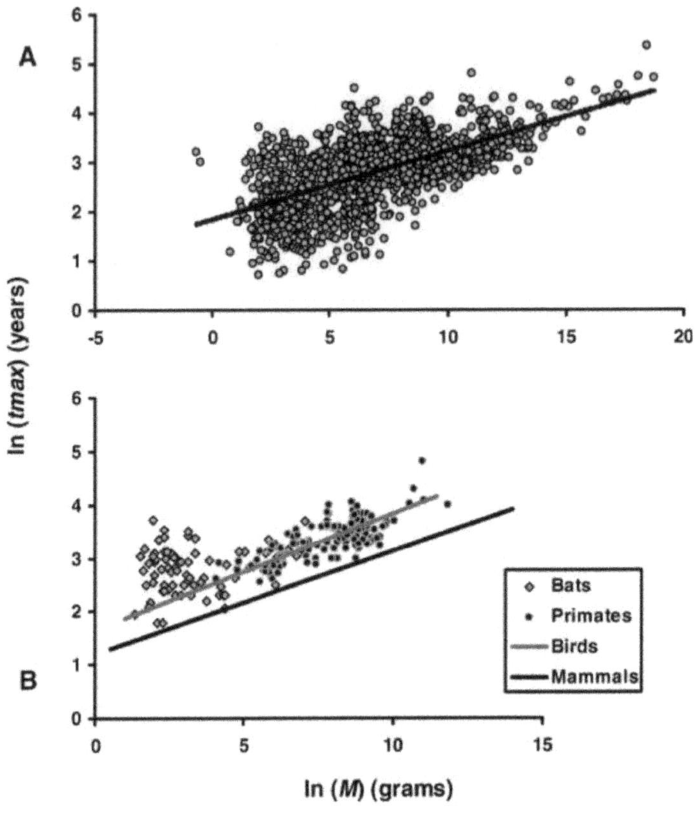

Fig.2

According to our theoretical model, the total number of cells in an animal remains constant after reaching adulthood. We assume that when the proportion of aging cells reaches a certain level δ of the total cell count, the animal dies. For an animal with a total cell count of M, the animal dies when the proportion of aging cells reaches δ. This can be expressed as:

$$F(\beta, t) = V_0 \left(e^{K_1 t} - \beta \frac{e^{K_1 t} e^{-K_2 t}}{1 + \beta e^{-K_2 t}} \right) = \delta M$$

The animal's lifespan, tmax = T(K1, K2, M, β), can be solved. Assuming that the damage coefficient, immune capacity, and immune capacity decline coefficient of each animal's cells are consistent, the lifespan of the animal is only related to the animal's volume. Additionally, the relationship between animal volume and lifespan follows a certain curve pattern.

$$V_0 \left(e^{K_1 t} - \beta \frac{e^{K_1 t} e^{-K_2 t}}{1 + \beta e^{-K_2 t}} \right)$$

Using the data from Fig.1, we can simulate the relationship between animal weight (consistent with volume) and lifespan, as shown in the graph below (Fig.3). This graph is highly consistent with the relationship between animal volume and lifespan calculated by de Magalhães et al. (Fig.2).

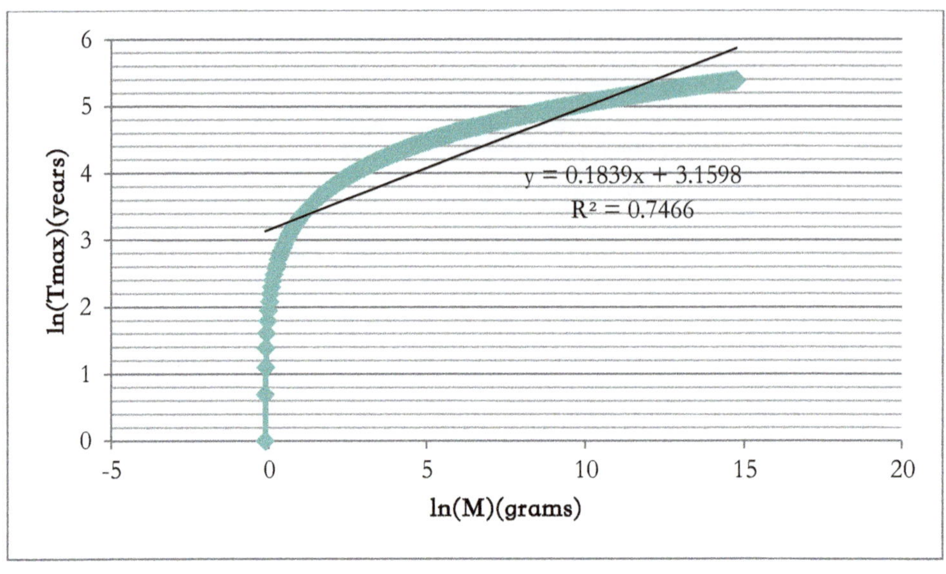

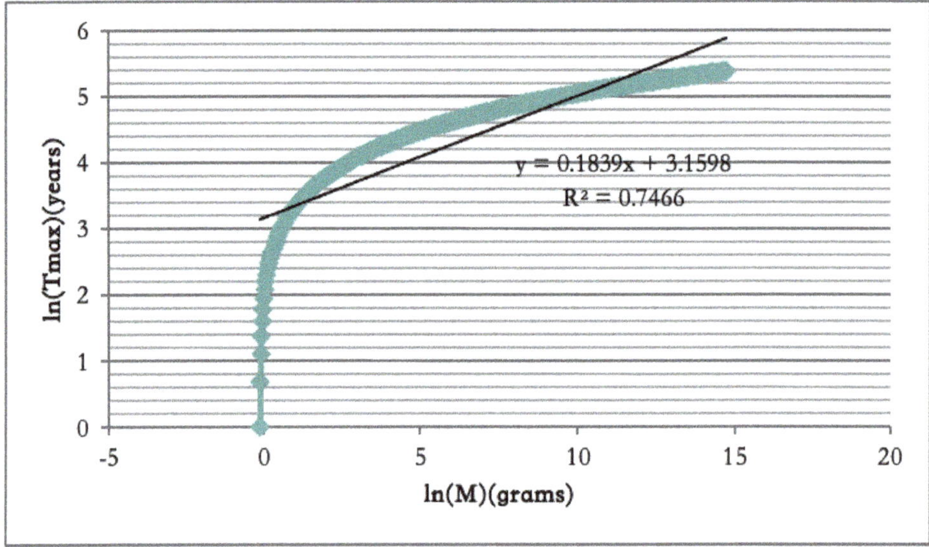

Fig.3

It is evident that explaining why larger animals have longer lifespans is straightforward in our model: as animal volume increases, the total number of cells in the animal after reaching adulthood also increases.

158

Consequently, a larger number of aging cells is required to cause the animal's death. The number of cells aging due to damage is only dependent on time. Therefore, with larger animal volumes, it takes longer to accumulate a certain proportion of aging cells, resulting in a longer lifespan for the animal.

2. Disease Treatment or Prevention

According to the laws of physics, when an animal falls ill, it indicates that some cells within the animal are in a dysfunctional state. The approach to treating diseases involves either repairing these cells (from bad to good) or directly removing them and replacing them with new cells. Taking humans as an example, when the body experiences a disease and some cells are inactive (functionally impaired) or deteriorated (harmful to the body), in our model, these cells are considered aging cells. So, how do we treat this disease? Physics dictates that we can only clear out these unfavorable cells (repairing a bad cell to a good cell at the cellular level is almost impossible for humans) and rely on the body's own mechanisms to regenerate normal cells from the remaining stem cells to replace the removed cells. Although our model does not explicitly include the process of stem cell regeneration, we assume that this process naturally occurs after the removal of bad cells. Stem cells regenerate into younger and healthier cells, and if this regeneration process occurs naturally and without other limiting factors, according to our model, once the removal of aging cells is completed, the rest will happen naturally. Here, we assume that this process occurs naturally.

Assuming a chronic disease such as diabetes, cancer, or Alzheimer's occurs, the accumulation of aging cells in patients increases following the blue curve in Fig.1. Without treatment, the patient is highly likely to die earlier than normal individuals. By employing an effective treatment method, the impact of treatment is reflected in the backward shift of the aging cell accumulation curve.

According to our model, there should be two types of treatment methods: 1) Direct removal of aging cells (green line in Fig.1); 2) Enhancing immune capacity, which can increase the clearance of aging cells through improved immunity (purple line in Fig.1). In any case, an effective treatment method will result in the aging cell accumulation curve shifting backward, causing the intersection point with the death line to move backward as well, essentially extending the patient's lifespan. Many treatment methods can both directly remove aging cells and enhance immune capacity (for instance, clearing aging cells may present antigens to the immune system, boosting the immune response to clear more aging cells, depicted by the red line in Fig.1), leading to a further backward shift of the aging cell curve and greater extension of lifespan.

In reality, examples such as tumor ablation to improve patient survival and extending animal lifespan through the removal of aging cells align with our model. In contrast to lethal cancers, the treatment of diabetes is more about prevention or reducing damage, as diabetes treatment doesn't seem to involve clearing aging cells. Instead, diabetes treatment often focuses on lowering blood sugar to limit further damage caused by high blood sugar to the body's systems. This approach may be related to the chronic nature of diabetes and the lack of effective means to cure diabetes.

3. Toxic Excitation Effects

Some treatment methods exhibit a unique pattern where substances that are generally toxic to the human body are introduced into the body. At low doses, these substances aid in the elimination of diseases, or in other words, low doses of "toxic" substances can trigger excitatory effects that benefit the body.

For example, in the past, it was widely believed that free radicals (ROS) induced oxidative stress, damaging normal cells in the body and potentially leading to the loss or transformation of these cells into cancer cells (similar to our unified theory's concept of aging cells). However, extensive use has revealed that, in essence, the generation of ROS in the body is generally beneficial. For instance, exercise can generate ROS, and it is well-established that exercise is beneficial for conditions like diabetes and cancer. Increasing ROS levels can even treat autoimmune diseases like arthritis. If we were to strictly adhere to the harmful effects of free radicals theory, one would assume that individuals should consume antioxidants daily to combat such damage. However, how do we explain the occurrence of these toxic excitation effects observed in reality?

Using our model, we can easily explain this. We determine the effectiveness of a treatment by observing whether it increases or decreases the presence of aging cells, in other words, whether it causes

$$\frac{dV}{dt} = K_1 V(1 - \rho(t, \ \beta)),$$

to increase or decrease. If it increases, we consider the treatment to be ineffective as it leads to an increase in aging cells. Conversely, if it decreases, we deem the treatment effective as it reduces the number of aging cells. The presence of free radicals increases oxidative stress on normal cells, but since this damage accumulates gradually over time at a steady pace, there shouldn't be significant fluctuations in the middle. The effects of artificially reducing free radical levels temporarily are not substantial. If we only consider this aspect, the theory of free radical damage remains valid. However, our model also includes $\rho(t, \beta)$, which represents the function of immune clearance capacity.

We also know that an essential tool of the immune system is ROS, where neutrophils and macrophages use ROS to clear various aging cells (such as infected cells or cancer cells) by increasing ROS levels and relying on their oxidative properties to eliminate these undesirable cells. While increasing ROS levels may damage normal cells, it also enhances the immune system's ability to clear aging cells. When the supplemented dose of ROS is low, such as the temporary increase in ROS levels in the body after exercise, it benefits the immune system in clearing aging cells, resulting in

$$\frac{dV}{dt} = K_1 V(1 - \rho(t, \ \beta)),$$

 decreasing. Overall, increasing ROS levels is advantageous for overall health.

Therefore, the toxic excitatory effect of free radicals relies on the short-term increase in free radicals to enhance the immune system's ability to clear aging cells, resulting in a greater reduction in the number of aging cells compared to the additional aging cells generated by the damage to normal cells caused by free radicals. This can be metaphorically described

$$\frac{dV}{dt} \downarrow = K_1 \uparrow V(1 - \rho(t, \ \beta) \downarrow)$$

as:

The short-term increase in free radicals leads to a decrease in $\frac{dV}{dt}$.

References:

1) de Magalhães, J. P., J. Costa, and G. M. Church. "An Analysis of the Relationship Between Metabolism, Developmental Schedules, and Longevity Using Phylogenetic Independent Contrasts." The Journals of Gerontology: Series A 62.2(2007):400–407.

2) BAKER D J, WIJSHAKE T, TCHKONIA T, et al. Clearance of p16Ink4a-positive senescent cells delays ageing-associated disorders. Nature, 2011, 479: 232-236.

3) Watson J D. Type 2 diabetes as a redox disease. Lancet 2014; 383(9919):841-3.

4) Hultqvist M, Olofsson P, Gelderman KA, Holmberg J, Holmdahl R. A New Arthritis Therapy with Oxidative Burst Inducers. PLoS Medicine 2006; 3(9):e348.

11. A PRECLINICAL RESEARCH REPORT

Intratumoral Delivery of Chlorine Dioxide Exploits its ROS-like Properties: A Novel Paradigm for Effective Cancer Therapy

Xuewu Liu[a]*, Zhaoyang Liu[b], Xueyan Liu[c], Shuangning Liu[d], Jiao Zhang[a]

[a] Beijing Wanbincell Biotechnology Co., Ltd., Wangjing Street, Chaoyang District, 100102, Beijing, China

[b] The Cancer Institute and Hospital, Chinese Academy of Medical Sciences, No. 17 Panjiayuan Nanli, Chaoyang District, 100021, Beijing, China

[c] The Third People's Hospital of Yinchuan, 128 Yuhuangge North Street, Xingqing District, Yinchuan, 750001, Ningxia, China

[d] International Department of Beijing No.80 High School, 16 Wangjing North Road, Chaoyang District,100102, Beijing, China

* Corresponding author. Email:liuxuewu@wanbincell.com

Highlights

- Chlorine dioxide: safe and effective, exhibits ROS-like properties for cancer elimination and tissue regeneration.
- Intratumoral delivery of chlorine dioxide: targets and eliminates cancer cells without promoting drug resistance.

- Chlorine dioxide stimulates an immune response against cancer, enhancing therapeutic potential.
- Intratumoral injections of chlorine dioxide: innovative strategy for effective cancer therapy.

Abstract

Reactive Oxygen Species (ROS) are potent oxidizing compounds renowned for their ability to eradicate cancer cells and facilitate tissue regeneration. In our research, we have discovered chlorine dioxide (CD), a substance that exhibits ROS-like properties and can be safely administered as a medicinal agent in the human body. Our study focuses on the utilization of intratumoral delivery of CD as a novel and efficacious approach for cancer therapy. Through intratumoral injections, CD selectively targets and eliminates cancer cells without promoting drug resistance. Furthermore, CD has demonstrated the capacity to elicit an immune response against cancer, thereby augmenting its therapeutic potential. We propose a groundbreaking paradigm for cancer treatment, employing intratumoral injections of CD, which holds great promise in prolonging the survival of cancer patients and transforming cancer into a manageable chronic condition. This approach harnesses the ROS-like properties of CD to effectively eradicate cancer cells while fostering tissue regeneration. By capitalizing on the unique characteristics of CD, we present a new avenue for enhancing patient outcomes in cancer therapy. Further research is warranted to optimize the administration protocols and dosage of CD, as well as to explore potential synergistic effects with other therapeutic agents. With ongoing investigation, the intratumoral delivery of CD represents a promising and innovative strategy for achieving effective cancer therapy.

Keywords

Reactive Oxygen Species, chlorine dioxide, cancer cells, tissue regeneration, intratumoral delivery, drug resistance, immune response.

Abbreviations

SOD- Superoxide dismutase

ROS - Reactive Oxygen Species

PDT - Photodynamic therapy

CD - Chlorine dioxide

DAMPs - Death-associated molecular patterns

HCMs - Human cardiac myocytes

HUVECs - Human vascular endothelial cells

NSCLC - non-small cell lung cancer

LT - Large tumor

ST - Small tumor

Introduction

Certain natural compounds or drugs that target Superoxide dismutase (SOD) possess a unique capability to selectively eradicate cancer cells by stimulating the generation or accumulation of Reactive Oxygen Species (ROS) [1, 2]. Furthermore, the body's neutrophils can also generate ROS, which contributes to the destruction of cancer cells [3]. Certain drugs can selectively enhance the levels of ROS in cancer cells, exhibiting long-term inhibitory effects on cancer. For example, the combination of metformin-induced ROS upregulation and apigenin amplification results in significant anticancer activity while preserving the integrity of normal cells [4]. Photodynamic therapy (PDT) is a treatment method that utilizes light to activate a photosensitizer within the body, resulting in the production of singlet oxygen ($^1O_2$). This sudden increase in oxygen levels induces toxicity in tumor cells, leading to their demise through apoptosis or necrosis. PDT not only directly targets and eradicates the tumor but also stimulates the release of cell death-associated molecular patterns (DAMPs) by dendritic cells, activating the immune system's antigen-presenting response and promoting an anti-tumor immune response [5].

Based on our hypothesis, we propose that the exogenous supplementation of ROS or their analogs could effectively eradicate tumors and, similar to PDT, elicit an antitumor immune response. In this study, we have selected chlorine dioxide (CD) as a ROS-like oxidant to evaluate its potential in cancer therapy. CD is widely acknowledged as a potent oxidizing agent with disinfectant properties, distinguished by its molecular formula ClO_2. Its applications encompass various domains, including water treatment, food processing, medical hygiene, and environmental cleaning. Notably, CD exhibits rapid destruction of cell membranes and DNA in bacteria, viruses, and other microorganisms, thereby effectively eliminating pathogens and contaminants. Remarkably, at lower concentrations of 0.25 mg/L, CD can eradicate 99% of E. coli (15,000 cells/mL) within a mere 15 seconds [6]. Furthermore, studies have demonstrated that CD and hydrogen peroxide demonstrate comparable efficacy in inducing cell death in human gingival fibroblasts [7].

ROS are generated during cellular respiration for ATP production [8]. However, the dispersed nature of ROS production in the body and the limited capacity to rapidly eliminate a large number of cells, especially within tumor tissues, present significant challenges. These challenges are primarily attributed to tumor hypoxia, characterized by low oxygen levels in the tumor microenvironment [9]. To establish a novel paradigm for cancer treatment, it is crucial to elevate the concentration of CD to a level that can effectively eradicate substantial tumor masses. This concentration exceeds the typical endogenous ROS production in the body. Furthermore, considering the short half-life of CD as an oxidizing agent in body tissues and the imperative of minimizing systemic side effects, intratumoral administration of CD has been selected as the preferred approach to achieve our objective.

Materials and methods

Cell Culture

An MTT assay was conducted to assess the inhibitory effect of a CD solution on the survival rate of MCF-7 breast cancer cells, human cardiac myocytes (HCM), and human vascular endothelial cells (HUVECs).

Additionally, the MTT assay was utilized to determine the survival inhibition rate of ten non-small cell lung cancer (NSCLC) cell lines, namely H2110, H1975, H650, H1623, H2126, HCC827, A549, H810, H1048, and H1355. To evaluate apoptosis or necrosis in MCF-7 breast cancer cells and human cardiac myocytes, flow cytometry with Annexin-V PI double staining was employed. The cells were incubated with varying concentrations of CD for 24 hours at 37°C, harvested, and washed with DMEM. Subsequently, the cells were resuspended in annexin V-FITC and PI staining solution, followed by a 15-minute incubation in the dark at room temperature. After the addition of binding buffer, the stained cells were analyzed using a FACSCalibur flow cytometer, with FITC fluorescence measured between 515 and 545 nm and PI fluorescence measured between 564 and 606 nm.

Reagent

CD solution at concentrations of 8mg/mL, 13mg/mL, and 15mg/mL was obtained from Beijing Wanbincell Biotechnology Co., Ltd.

Animal Models

C57BL/6 and Balb/c mice were obtained from the China Experimental Center for Food, Drugs, and Biological Products. All experiments were conducted with the approval of the The Cancer Institute and Hospital, Chinese Academy of Medical Sciences.

Mouse Safety Studies

C57BL/6 mice were administered a single intraperitoneal injection of 0.3 mL of a CD solution (7.5 mg/mL), which was determined to be well-tolerated. Similarly, a single dose of 0.5 mL of a CD solution (1 mg/mL) was found to be safe for C57BL/6 mice. However, when a single dose of 0.2 mL of a CD solution (7.5 mg/mL) was injected into the caudal vein, tail loss was observed at the injection site, potentially due to CD-induced damage to blood vessels and subsequent ischemic necrosis. On the other hand, intracranial injection of a single dose of 0.02 mL of a CD solution (1.5 mg/mL) was deemed safe for C57BL/6 mice.

CD simulated the impact of ROS on healthy tissues.

Two groups of female C57BL/6 mice, aged 9-10 weeks, were randomly assigned into two groups, with each group consisting of four mice (n=4). The first group received a subcutaneous injection of 0.3 mL of a CD solution with a concentration of 7.5 mg/mL, while the second group received a subcutaneous injection of 0.3 mL of a CD solution with a concentration of 15 mg/mL. The injection sites were monitored daily, and the extent of injury was assessed and recorded using an injury score. The injury score was determined by multiplying the area of the lesion by the severity of the lesion.

Effect of CD on Tissue Regeneration in Mice

Twenty female C57BL/6 mice (9-10 weeks old) were anesthetized with halothane and had their tails severed 2 cm from the base. The mice were randomly divided into 5 groups, each consisting of 4 mice. Group 1 immersed their tail wounds in a 15mg/mL CD solution for 1 minute and received daily treatment with the same solution. Group 2 immersed their tail wounds in physiological saline solution for 1 minute and received daily treatment with the same solution. Group 3 immersed their tail wounds in a 15mg/mL CD solution for 10 minutes daily for 8 consecutive days, and then on days 10, 14, and 18. Group 4 immersed their tail wounds in a 1.5% hydrogen peroxide solution for 10 minutes daily for 8 consecutive days, and then on days 10, 14, and 18. The progress of wound healing and tail severance wound scores were recorded. Group 5 immersed their tail wounds in a 15mg/mL CD solution for 10 minutes on days 1, 4, 8, 12, 16, and 20. Wound healing progress was assessed using a scale ranging from 0 (fully healed) to 90 (exudate or crusting area).

Inhibition of Lewis Lung Cancer in Mice by Intrapericardial Injection of CD Solution

A total of ten male C57BL/6 mice, aged 9-10 weeks, were included in the study. The mice were subcutaneously inoculated with 4×10^6 LLC cells in the right axillary region and subsequently divided into two groups, with ten mice in each group. Starting from the 4th day after cell inoculation, the CD solution was intratumorally injected at a dosage of 0.2mL per mouse (8 mg/mL) every other day for a total of three doses. From the second injection onwards, the dosage was increased to 0.3mL per mouse. The control group received intratumoral injections of PBS injection solution. The experimental period lasted for 10 days, after which all animals were humanely euthanized two days following the administration of the final dose in the experimental group. Tumor weight was measured after recording the animals' body weight, and the tumor suppression rate was calculated. Tumor length and width were regularly measured to accurately calculate tumor volume.

Inhibition of B16 Melanoma Growth in C57BL/6 Mice by Intratumoral Injection of CD Solution.

Each male C57BL/6 mouse, aged 9-10 weeks, was subcutaneously inoculated with 2×10^6 cells in the right axillary region. Subsequently, the mice were randomly divided into three groups, with ten mice in each group. On the 8th day after the inoculation of B16 cancer cells, the intratumoral injection group received CD solution intratumorally. The CD solution was administered at a dosage of 0.2mL (13mg/mL) every 4 days for a total of three doses. On the 2nd day after the inoculation of melanoma, the mouse tail vein injection group received CD solution via the tail vein. The CD solution was injected at a dosage of 0.2mL (1.5 mg/mL) every 4 days for a total of five doses. The tumor model group served as the control and received intratumoral injections of PBS injection solution for observation purposes. The experiment was conducted over a period of 20 days. Four animals from each group were humanely euthanized four days after the last dose, and their tumor weight was measured after recording their body weight in order to calculate the tumor suppression rate. On the 20th day, the remaining mice in each group were tested for cytokines.

Inhibition of Melanoma B16 Metastasis in C57BL/6 Mice by CD Solution.

Each male C57BL/6 mouse, aged 9-10 weeks, was subcutaneously inoculated with 2×10^6 B16 cells in the right axillary region and 1×10^6 B16 cells in the tail vein. Subsequently, the mice were randomly divided into three groups, with 9 mice in each group. The groups consisted of a tumor model control group, which received intratumoral injections of PBS solution; an intratumoral administration group in the axillary region; and an intratumoral administration group in the axillary region with daily 2-hour inhalation treatment for the tumor-bearing mice.

The administration of CD solution began on the 7th day after melanoma inoculation. The intratumoral injections of CD solution were administered at a volume of 0.2mL (15 mg/mL) every 4 days for a total of 4 doses. In the inhalation group, the mice received intratumoral injections of CD solution at the same dosage and frequency, along with 2 hours of daily inhalation treatment. For the inhalation treatment, 20mL of 15 mg/mL CD solution was placed in the mouse cage for natural evaporation and inhalation.

On the 17th day, three mice from each group underwent HE staining of the tumor tissue and lungs. On the 21st day, the lungs were harvested, and the pulmonary metastatic foci were counted.

Inhibitory Effect of Intratumoral CD Solution on 4T1 Breast Cancer Cell Transplantation in Balb/c Mice

A total of 32 female Balb/c mice, aged 9-10 weeks, were utilized for this experiment. They were divided into four groups, each consisting of eight mice. The large tumor group (LT group) received a subcutaneous inoculation of 4×10^5 4T1 cells in the right axillary region and contralateral mammary pad. Subsequently, they were randomly assigned to two groups: the control group (PBS+LT) and the treatment group (CD+LT), with eight mice in each group. Similarly, the small tumor group (ST group) received a subcutaneous inoculation of 2×10^5 4T1 cells in the right axillary region and contralateral mammary pad. They were then divided into the control group (PBS+ST) and the treatment group (CD+ST), with eight mice in each group.

Starting from the 15th day after inoculation, groups 2 and 4 (CD+LT and CD+ST) received intratumoral injections of a CD solution with a concentration of 15 mg/mL. A total volume of 0.2 mL (15 mg/mL) was administered every 3 days for a total of 6 doses. The mammary pad tumors in the control groups (PBS+LT and PBS+ST) were observed without any treatment (Untreated). On the 27th day, partial immune cells were tested, and on the 33rd day, the animals were euthanized. The lungs were harvested for counting pulmonary metastasis, as well as for the detection of serum and axillary tumor cytokines.

On the 27th day of the 4T1 model, blood and spleen samples were collected from 3 mice in each group, totaling 12 mice. Whole blood samples were collected from 12 mice, and spleen samples were collected from the remaining 12 mice. The spleen suspended cells were prepared for the detection of CD3, CD4, CD8, and CD335 using four-color staining, as well as CD11b, Gr-1, and F4/80 using three-color staining. Fresh anticoagulated peripheral blood from the mice (spleen suspended cells) was added to the bottom of the flow cytometry sample tube, and an appropriate amount of fluorescently labeled antibodies was added, including CD3e PerCP-Cy5.5, CD4 PE, CD8a FITC, and CD335 (NKp46) APC (Biolegend), as well as Gr-1 FITC, F4/80 PE, and CD11b APC (Biolegend). Analysis was performed using a flow cytometer (BD).

On the 33rd day of the 4T1 model, blood and axillary tumor samples were collected from 5 mice in each group, totaling 20 mice (Untreated). ELISA was used to measure the levels of IL-6, TNF-α, INF-γ, and CTLA-4 in the serum and tumor samples.

Statistics

Statistical analyses were performed using Origin 9.0 software. When the transformed data showed significant variation among treatments, differences among populations and treatments were assessed using the nonparametric Mann-Whitney test. However, in most cases, no significant variation was observed among treatments. In such instances, two-tailed Student's t-tests were used to evaluate differences between two treatments. For comparisons involving more than two treatments, a two-way ANOVA followed by Dunnett's multiple comparisons tests was employed to compare multiple groups with repeated measures.

Results and Discussion

Our initial safety experiment confirmed the safe administration of the CD solution at various concentrations to the mice in this study. CD exhibits potent cytotoxicity against breast cancer cells as well as normal cells, including cardiomyocytes and vascular endothelial cells (Fig. 1A, B). It induces cell death through both apoptotic and necrotic pathways, similar to ROS, which can trigger cell death through necrotic or apoptotic mechanisms [10], regardless of the cell type (Fig. 1C).

Due to the non-selective cytotoxicity of CD towards the cells it encounters, systemic administration of CD as a drug is not feasible. Therefore, intratumoral administration is a suitable choice for targeting solid tumors. In our study, we administered CD via subcutaneous injection in the dorsal region of mice, and the results revealed significant damage to normal tissues caused by CD. Injection of CD resulted in severe skin damage in mice and noticeable necrosis of various cell types in the subcutaneous tissue. However, approximately 20 days later, the damaged tissue completely recovered, and the skin returned to its original state (Fig. 2A, B), with successful hair regrowth (Supplementary Fig. S1D). This indicates that the tissue damage caused by CD is not cumulative and that the damaged tissue is capable of complete regeneration.

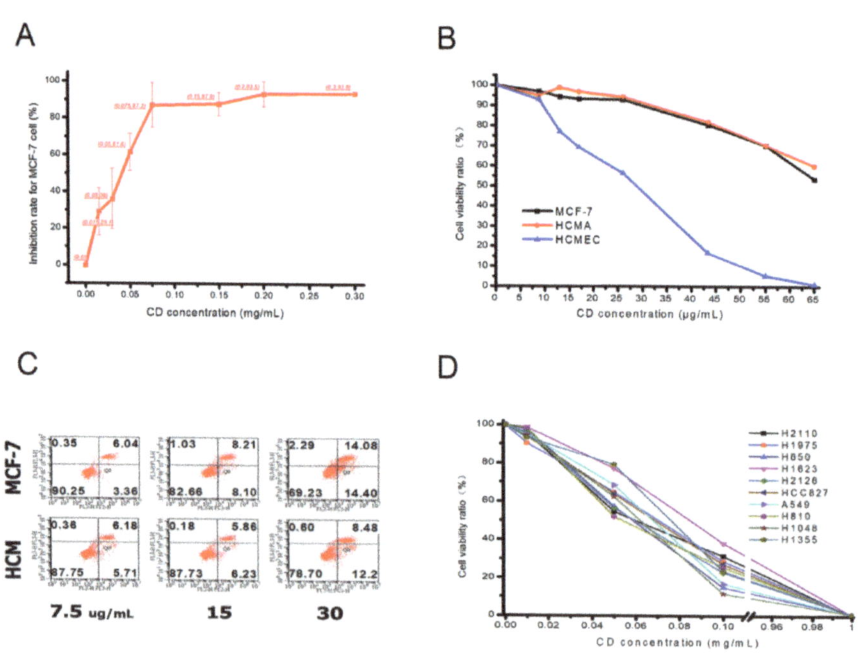

Fig. 1. In vitro cell viability assay of CD. (A) Inhibition of cell survival in MCF-7 human breast cancer cells by CD. (B) Percentage of cell survival inhibition by CD in MCF-7 breast cancer cells, normal human cardiomyocytes (HCM), and human vascular endothelial cells (HCMEA). (C) Representative plots demonstrating the measurement of apoptosis or necrotic pathways in breast cancer cells and cardiomyocytes using flow cytometry after treatment with different concentrations of CD (The lower right quadrant represents early apoptotic cells, and the upper right quadrant represents necrotic or late apoptotic cells). (D) Measurement of cell proliferation in 10 NSCLC cell lines when treated with increasing doses of CD.

Neutrophils have the ability to produce hypochlorous acid, an oxidizing agent similar to ROS, which has been demonstrated to accelerate skin wound healing and promote skin rejuvenation when applied topically [11]. Similarly, hydrogen peroxide, another type of ROS, has been found to facilitate sensory axon regeneration in zebrafish skin [12]. Building upon these findings, we formulated the hypothesis that CD may also possess the capability to promote tissue regeneration. To investigate this hypothesis, we applied CD to wounds created by cutting the tails of mice. Remarkably, both CD treatment and hydrogen peroxide treatment significantly expedited the healing process in tail-ablated mice compared to treatment with physiological saline, resulting in complete wound closure approximately 6 days earlier (Supplementary Fig. S1A-B, E). Prolonged exposure to the CD solution in one group led to significant damage to the excised wound and the surrounding normal skin tissue. However, once the exposure was reduced, the damaged skin rapidly regenerated without impeding the healing of the original wound (Supplementary Fig. S1C). As an oxidant, CD also facilitated the oxidation of cellular tissue debris, thereby promoting the clearance of deposits near the wound (Supplementary Fig. S1F). This mechanism may potentially serve as a pathway for tissue regeneration..

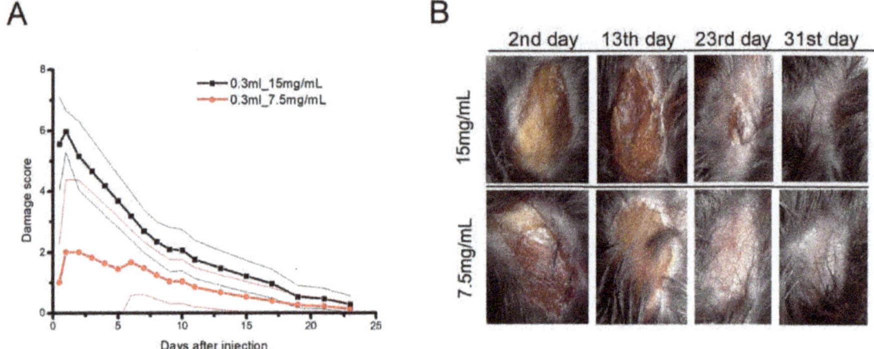

Fig. 2. In vivo tissue damage and regeneration assay of CD. (A) Injection of CD solution at concentrations of 15mg/mL and 7.5mg/mL subcutaneously into the dorsal region of C57BL/6 mice, showing the trend of injury scores (injury recovery) over time. Data presented as mean ± SD (n=4). (B) Representative images of the back skin taken on days 2, 13, and 23 after the start of CD injection. Images selected from each group.

On the fourth day following subcutaneous inoculation of LLC cancer cells in C57BL/6 mice, we initiated intratumoral injection of a lower dose (8mg/mL) of CD. Notably, compared to the control group, the intratumoral injection of CD on the sixth day exhibited a substantial suppression of tumor growth (Fig. 3A; Supplementary Fig. S2B). Furthermore, the CD-injected tumors displayed evident necrosis, indicating a robust necrotic effect on the tumor tissue (Supplementary Fig. S2A). To further investigate the therapeutic potential of CD, we escalated the dosage to 13 mg/mL and additionally employed intravenous injection at a concentration of 1.5 mg/mL in a B16 tumor model. Remarkably, the intratumoral injection group demonstrated significant tumor suppression (74.1% inhibition) on day 4, while the intravenous group exhibited a comparatively weaker but still significant inhibition (34.8% inhibition). Subsequent evaluations revealed that the intratumoral injection group consistently exhibited a higher degree of tumor suppression, whereas the intravenous group failed to exhibit any inhibitory effect (Fig. 3B). Intravenous administration of CD resulted in a reduced tumor burden, suggesting a potential involvement of antitumor immunity, albeit without sustained efficacy. On day 20, IL-1β and VEGF levels were assessed in the mice, revealing no significant differences between the groups (Supplementary Fig. S3A, B).

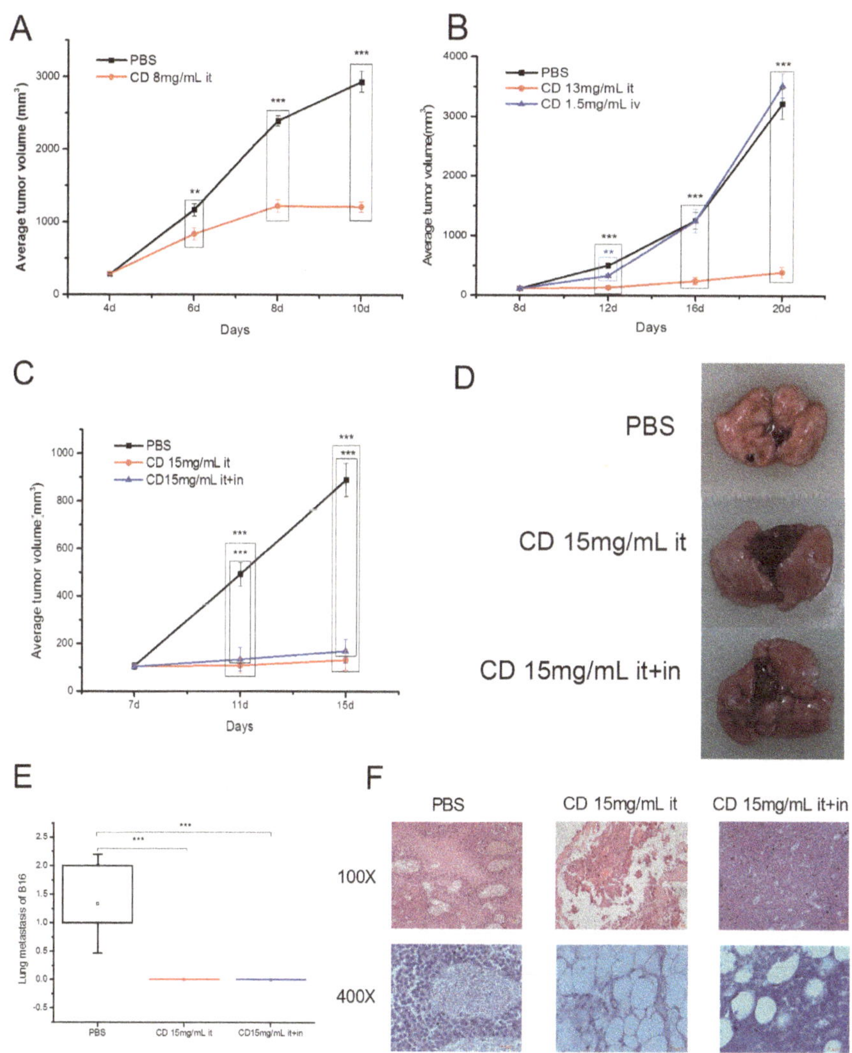

Fig. 3. In vivo anti-cancer assay of CD through intratumoral injection in C57BL/6 mice. (A) Subcutaneous tumor volume of LLC cancer cells. One group received intratumoral injection of PBS as a control, while another group received intratumoral injection of CD (8mg/mL). (**P < 0.01, *** P < 0.001, two-tailed t-test; n = 10 mice per cohort). Error bars represent mean ± SEM. (B) Subcutaneous tumor volume of B16 cells, with one group receiving intratumoral injection of PBS as a control, another group receiving intratumoral injection of CD (13 mg/mL), and a third group receiving intravenous injection of CD (1.5 mg/mL). (**P < 0.01, *** P < 0.001, two-tailed t-test; n = 10 mice per cohort). Error bars represent mean ± SEM. (C) Tumor volume of subcutaneous and lung metastasis models established by subcutaneous and tail vein injection of B16 cells, with one group receiving intratumoral injection of PBS, another group receiving intratumoral injection of CD (15 mg/mL), and a third group receiving intratumoral injection of CD (15mg/mL) along with daily inhalation of CD gas. (*** P < 0.001, two-tailed t-test; n = 9 mice per cohort). Error bars represent mean ± SEM. (D) Lung metastasis nodules counted on day 21 in the subcutaneous and lung metastasis models. (E) Lung metastasis nodules counted on day 21. (*** P < 0.001, two-tailed t-test; n = 3 mice per cohort). Error bars represent mean ± SD. (F) Histological images of subcutaneous and lung metastasis models on day 17 stained with H&E (100x and 400x magnification).

In the context of cancer cell death, both apoptosis and necrosis have been shown to elicit anti-cancer immune responses [13, 14]. Based on this knowledge, we hypothesized that direct injection of CD into tumors could induce apoptosis and necrosis of cancer cells, thereby activating the body's anti-tumor immune response. To investigate this hypothesis, we established B16 tumor and B16 lung metastasis models in C57BL/6 mice. Our findings revealed that CD significantly inhibited tumor progression, while daily inhalation of CD gas had minimal impact on subcutaneous tumors (Fig. 3C). On day 21, the mice's lungs were examined to assess the presence of B16 lung metastases. In the control group, each mouse (n=3) exhibited 1-2 lung metastatic foci. However, in both the intratumoral injection of CD and the combination of intratumoral injection and inhalation of CD gas groups (n=5), no lung metastatic foci were observed (Fig. 3D). These results indicate that intratumoral CD injection can directly ablate the tumor and trigger a systemic anti-tumor immune response, leading to significant inhibition of tumor metastasis (Fig. 3E).

Histological analysis on the 17th day revealed extensive necrotic centers and destruction of the tumor architecture following CD injection (Fig. 3F). Although inhalation of CD gas caused some lung damage (Supplementary Fig. S4), it did not affect B16 lung metastasis.

In our study, we utilized a mouse model and injected 4T1 tumor cells into the mammary pad and axillary regions of BALB/c mice. Two groups of mice were administered different concentrations of tumor cells: a small tumor group (ST) received 4×105 cells in the mammary pad and 2×105 cells in the axillary region, while a large tumor group (LT) received 4×105 cells in both regions. On the 15th day, CD (15 mg/mL) was administered exclusively into the mammary pad tumors of the experimental group. We observed a significant reduction in tumor volume in the CD-treated groups, particularly in the small tumor group (P < 0.05) (Fig. 4A, B). The large tumor group exhibited a 30% inhibition rate on the third day, whereas the small tumor group demonstrated a higher inhibition rate of 72%. The axillary tumors displayed a lower tumor suppression rate due to the absence of direct killing effects from CD. However, at 21 and 27 days, the CD-treated groups exhibited significantly higher inhibition rates compared to the control groups (Fig. 4C, D). These findings suggest that intratumoral CD injection can induce an anti-tumor immune response, although the response may not be sustained. T-cell exhaustion is frequently observed in cancer [15], indicating a general decline in the immune system's ability to combat tumors under various circumstances. On the 27th and 33rd days, lung metastasis was significantly inhibited in the CD-treated groups compared to the control groups. The small tumor group exhibited a slightly delayed response compared to the large tumor group, but the difference was not statistically significant (Fig. 4E, G). These results underscore the potential of intratumoral CD injection as a therapeutic strategy for inhibiting tumor growth and metastasis.

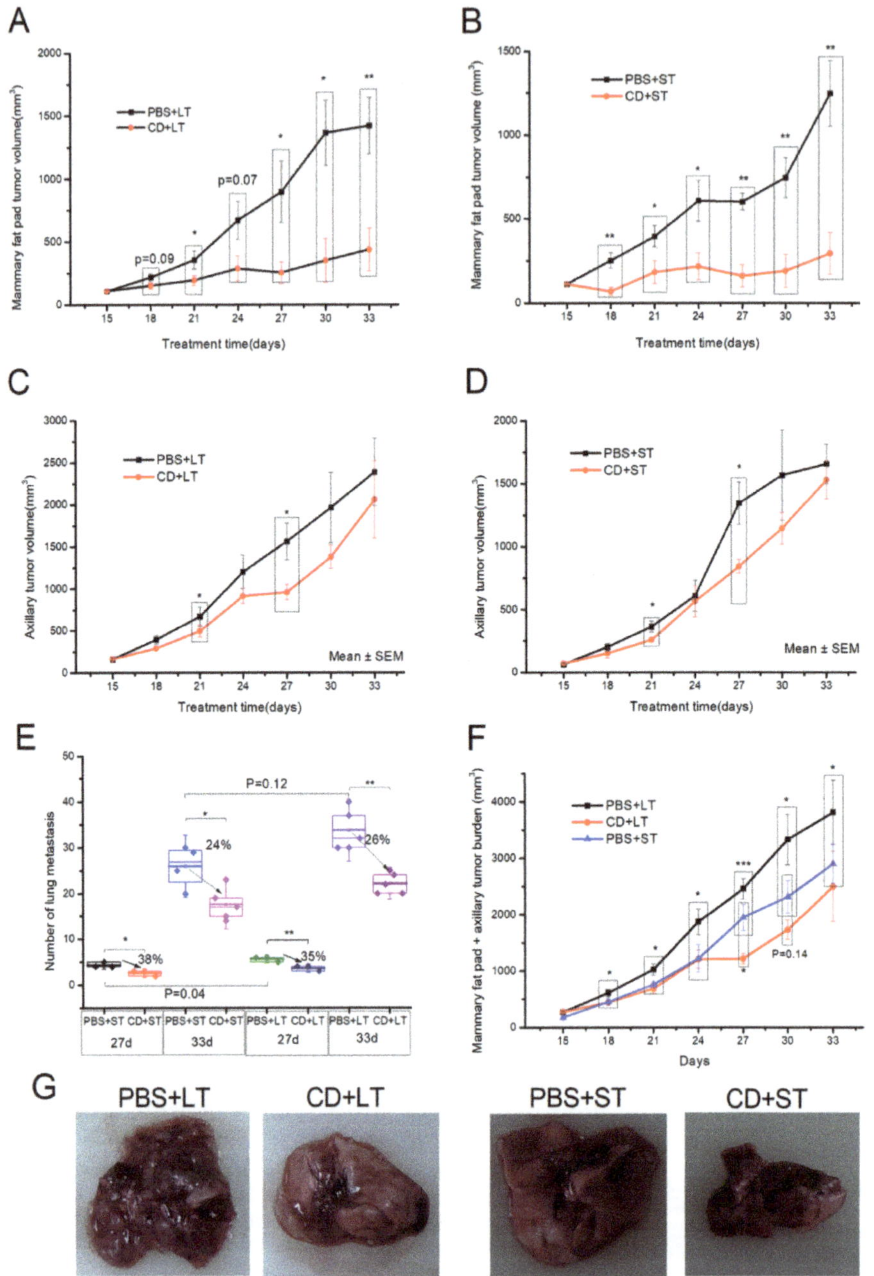

Fig. 4. **In vivo anti-cancer assay of CD through intratumoral injection in BALB/c mice.** (A) Schematic representation of the subcutaneous and mammary pad injection of 4T1 tumor cells and the administration of CD. (B) Tumor volume

of the large tumor group, with one group receiving intratumoral injection of PBS as a control (PBS+LT) and another group receiving intratumoral injection of CD (15 mg/mL) as a treatment (CD+LT). (*P < 0.05, ** P < 0.01, two-tailed t-test; n = 5-8 mice per cohort). Error bars represent mean ± SEM. (C) Tumor volume of the small tumor group, with one group receiving intratumoral injection of PBS as a control (PBS+ST) and another group receiving intratumoral injection of CD (15 mg/mL) as a treatment (CD+ST). (*P < 0.05, ** P < 0.01, two-tailed t-test; n = 4-8 mice per cohort). Error bars represent mean ± SEM. (D) Tumor volume of the large tumor group in the axilla (no injection). (*P < 0.05, two-tailed t-test; n = 5-8 mice per cohort). Error bars represent mean ± SEM. (E) Tumor volume of the small tumor group in the axilla (no injection). (*P < 0.05, two-tailed t-test; n = 4-8 mice per cohort). Error bars represent mean ± SEM. (F) Overall tumor burden, with the tumor volume of the large tumor group (mammary pad tumor injected with PBS) in the axilla added to represent the tumor burden of the control group, the tumor volume of the large tumor group (mammary pad tumor injected with CD) in the axilla added to represent the tumor burden of the treatment group, and the tumor volume of the small tumor group (mammary pad tumor injected with PBS) in the axilla added to represent the tumor burden of the control group. (*P < 0.05, ***P < 0.001, ANOVA, n = 5-8 mice per cohort). Error bars represent mean ± SEM. (G) Lung metastasis images on day 33, with the number of lung metastatic nodules roughly following the order: PBS+LT > CD+LT ≤ PBS+ST > CD+ST.

The presence of a primary tumor has been shown to decrease immunocompetence, but this can be improved by surgical resection of the primary tumor [16]. In our study, we investigated the effects of intratumoral CD injection for tumor ablation on the growth trajectory of tumors in different sizes. We hypothesized that if intratumoral CD injection can enhance the antitumor immune response, it would result in a significantly lower growth curve in the large tumor treatment group compared to the untreated growth curve of the small tumor group. To assess the overall tumor burden, we combined the mammary pad tumor and axillary tumor measurements. Our results showed that from day 24, the growth curve of the overall tumor burden in the large tumor treatment group deviated from that of the small tumor control group, with a notably lower growth rate. This suggests that intratumoral CD injection not only directly ablates the tumor and restores the dominant immune capability, but also provides additional immune enhancement. However, it is important to note that the immune enhancement observed was transient, as the growth curves of both groups started to converge after 30 days (Fig. 4F). These findings indicate that intratumoral CD injection has the potential to enhance the immune response against tumors, but further studies are needed to understand the duration and sustainability of this immune enhancement.

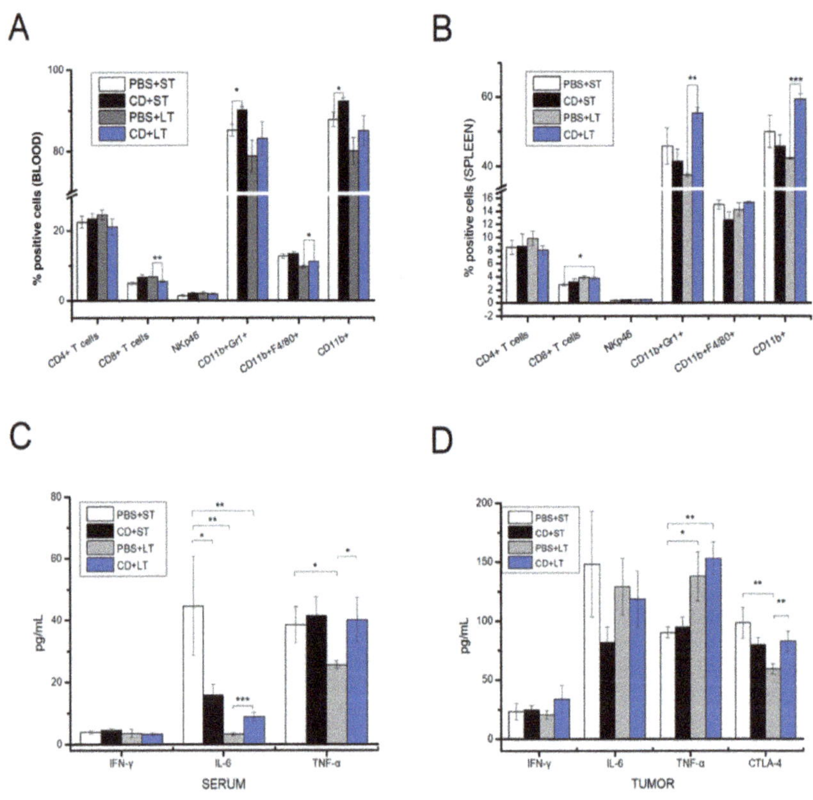

Fig. 5. Comprehensive analysis of the therapeutic effects of intratumoral CD injections in BLAB/c mice inoculated with 4T1 cells. (A) Flow cytometric analysis of plasma samples from mice at day 27, demonstrating quantification of CD4, CD8, NKp46, CD11b+Gr-1+, CD11b+F4/80+, and CD11b+ positive cells. (B) Flow cytometric analysis of spleen samples from mice at day 27, showing quantification of CD4, CD8, NKp46, CD11b+Gr-1+, CD11b+F4/80+, and CD11b+ positive cells. (C) Cytokine analysis of serum samples from mice at day

33. (D) Cytokine analysis of tumor samples from mice at day 33. (A-D) Data are presented as the mean ± SEM. Differences between therapy groups were assessed using two-way ANOVA followed by Dunnett's multiple comparisons tests (B-C: n=3; D-E: n=5).

On day 27, no significant changes were observed in CD4+ T cells and NKp46 cells in the plasma and spleen. However, the treatment group showed a significant increase in CD11b+Gr-1+ myeloid cells compared to the control group (Fig. 5A, B). In the large tumor group, the treatment group exhibited a significant decrease in CD8+ T cells in the plasma compared to the control group. Conversely, in the spleen, the treatment group in the large tumor group demonstrated a significant increase in CD8+ T cells compared to the control group in the small tumor group. These findings are consistent with the enhanced immune response induced by intratumoral CD injection. It is worth noting that CD11b+Gr-1+ cells possess immunosuppressive properties and contribute to the promotion of cancer metastasis [17], which may explain the transient nature of the immune response stimulated by intratumoral CD injection.

On day 33, cytokine levels in the serum and axillary tumors were evaluated. In the serum, a significant difference in TNF-α levels was observed between the large tumor group and the small tumor group. TNF-α levels increased during the later stages of tumor development, indicating that the antitumor immune response does not decline entirely but continues to rise, albeit at a relatively diminished rate compared to tumor evasion. The decrease in CTLA-4 levels also supports this observation. In the large tumor group, TNF-α levels significantly increased after treatment compared to the control group, consistent with the immune response triggered by intratumoral CD injection (Fig. 5C). Within the large tumor group, treatment with intratumoral CD injection led to a significant increase in CTLA-4 levels, potentially indicating a further reduction in immune capability. Regarding tumor tissue, the changes in TNF-α mirrored those observed in serum TNF-α (Fig. 5D). The alterations in IL-6 also correlated with TNF-α, suggesting potential interaction effects. The absolute value of immune capability in the large tumor group (both control and treatment) surpassed that of the preceding small tumor group. Following treatment in the large tumor group, the relative decrease in IL-6 compared to the control group in the small tumor group may be attributed to the additional immune response stimulated by intratumoral CD injection.

Conclusion

Our study highlights the potential of CD as a versatile therapeutic agent in cancer treatment. CD exhibits properties similar to ROS, such as promoting tissue regeneration and performing comparable functions. Considering the significant role of injury-induced ROS production in tissue regeneration [18], we have confirmed that CD can facilitate tissue regeneration in injured areas, akin to the role of ROS. Tumors can be regarded as non-healing wounds [19], presenting an opportunity to harness CD's regenerative capabilities during cancer treatment to expedite wound healing and enhance patient outcomes.

Compared to conventional cancer treatment methods, CD treatment offers numerous advantages. It significantly reduces disease complications and associated risks, providing a safer and more efficacious alternative. We propose the concept of intratumoral injection of CD, which involves direct tumor ablation without encountering resistance, while concurrently enhancing antitumor immunity. This approach minimizes harm to healthy tissues while harnessing the regenerative potential following tumor ablation. By embracing this comprehensive strategy, we can optimize the outcomes of cancer treatment.

In the future, as technology advances, the intratumoral administration of CD holds promise as a convenient and efficient approach in cancer treatment, reducing the burden on patients and potentially prolonging survival. This approach has the potential to transform cancer management into a chronic disease-like approach. Further research is needed to optimize administration protocols and dosage of CD, explore potential synergistic effects with other therapeutics, and elucidate its underlying mechanisms of regenerative and ablative effects on tumor tissue, as well as its ability to stimulate a systemic anti-tumor immune response. Ongoing research on CD demonstrates its potential as a valuable tool in cancer treatment, offering new possibilities for improved patient care and outcomes.

Author contributions

Xuewu Liu developed and designed the research framework, while Zhaoyang Liu, Xuewu Liu, Jiao Zhang, and Xueyan Liu carried out all the experiments. Xuewu Liu, Shuangning Liu, and Jiao Zhang analyzed the experimental data and drafted the manuscript. Shuangning Liu created the main figures. All authors have reviewed and approved the final version of the manuscript for publication.

Funding

This research did not receive any specific grant from funding agencies in the public, commercial, or not-for-profit sectors.

Declaration of competing interest

Xuewu Liu is the founder and owner of Beijing Wanbincell Biotechnology Co., Ltd. Jiao Zhang is an employee of Beijing Wanbincell Biotechnology Co., Ltd. Xuewu Liu. and Xueyan Liu are inventors on patent applications (WO2016074203 (A1) and WO2017152718 (A1)) filed by Xuewu Liu related to the use of chlorine dioxide for cancer treatment.

Appendix A. Supplementary (Omitted)

References

[1] Trachootham D, Zhou Y, Zhang H, Demizu Y, Chen Z, et al. Selective killing of oncogenically transformed cells through a ROS-mediated mechanism by beta-phenylethyl isothiocyanate. Cancer Cell. 10 (2006): 241–252. doi: 10.1016/j.ccr.2006.08.009

[2] Huang, P et al. "Superoxide dismutase as a target for the selective killing of cancer cells." Nature vol. 407,6802 (2000): 390-5. doi:10.1038/35030140

[3] Lichtenstein A, Seelig M, Berek J, Zighelboim J. Human neutrophil-mediated lysis of ovarian cancer cells. Blood 74 (1989): 805–809. doi: 10.1182/blood.V74.2.805.805

[4] Warkad, M.S., Kim, CH., Kang, BG. et al. Metformin-induced ROS upregulation as amplified by apigenin causes profound anticancer activity while sparing normal cells. Sci Rep 11, 14002 (2021). doi: 10.1038/s41598-021-93270-0

[5] Agostinis P, Berg K, Cengel KA, Foster TH, Girotti AW, et al. Photodynamic therapy of cancer: an update. CA Cancer J Clin. 61 (2011): 250–281. doi: 10.3322/caac.20114

[6] Benarde MA, Israel BM, Olivieri VP, Granstrom ML. Efficiency of Chlorine Dioxide as a Bactericide. Appl Microbiol. 13(5) (1965): 776–780. doi: 10.1128/AM.13.5.776-780.1965

[7] Nishikiori R, Nomura Y, Sawajiri M, Masuki K, Hirata I, Okazaki M. Influence of chlorine dioxide on cell death and cell cycle of human gingival fibroblasts. J Dent. 2008;36(12):993-998. doi:10.1016/j.jdent.2008.08.006

[8] Oka S, Tsuzuki T, Hidaka M, et al. Endogenous ROS production in early differentiation state suppresses endoderm differentiation via transient FOXC1 expression. Cell Death Discov. 8: 150 (2022). doi: 10.1038/s41420-022-00961-2

[9] Singleton DC, Macann A, Wilson WR. Therapeutic targeting of the hypoxic tumour microenvironment. Nat Rev Clin Oncol 18(2021): 751–772. doi: 10.1038/s41571-021-00539-4

[10] Ryter SW, Kim HP, Hoetzel A, Park JW, Nakahira K, Wang X, Choi AM. Mechanisms of cell death in oxidative stress. Antioxid Redox Signal. Jan;9(1) (2007):49-89. doi: 10.1089/ars.2007.9.49

[11] Leung TH, Zhang LF, Wang J, Ning S, Knox SJ, Kim SK. Topical hypochlorite ameliorates NF-κB-mediated skin diseases in mice. J Clin Invest. 123(2013): 5361–5370. doi: 10.1172/JCI70895

[12] Rieger S, Sagasti A. Hydrogen peroxide promotes injury-induced peripheral sensory axon regeneration in the zebrafish skin. PLoS Biol 9: e1000621 (2011). doi: 10.1371/journal.pbio.1000621

[13] Casares N, Pequignot MO, Tesniere A, Ghiringhelli F, Roux S, et al. Caspase-dependent immunogenicity of doxorubicin-induced tumor cell death. J Exp Med 202(2005): 1691–1701. doi: 10.1084/jem.20050915

[14] Aaes TL, Kaczmarek A, Delvaeye T, De Craene B, De Koker S, et al. Vaccination with Necroptotic Cancer Cells Induces Efficient Anti-tumor Immunity. Cell reports vol. 15,2 (2016): 274-87. doi: 10.1016/j.celrep.2016.03.037

[15] Wherry EJ, Kurachi M. Molecular and cellular insights into T-cell exhaustion. Nat Rev Immunol 15(8): 486–499 (2015). doi: 10.1038/nri3862

[16] Danna EA, Sinha P, Gilbert M, Clements VK, Pulaski BA, et al. Surgical removal of primary tumor reverses tumor-induced immunosuppression despite the presence of metastatic disease. Cancer Res 64(6) (2004): 2205-11. doi: 10.1158/0008-5472.can-03-2646

[17] Yan HH, Pickup M, Pang Y, Gorska AE, Li Z, et al. Gr-1+CD11b+ myeloid cells tip the balance of immune protection to tumor promotion in the premetastatic lung. Cancer Res 70(2010): 6139–6149. doi: 10.1158/0008-5472.CAN-10-0706

[18] Love NR, Chen Y, Ishibashi S, Kritsiligkou P, Lea R, et al. Amputation-induced reactive oxygen species are needed for successful Xenopus tadpole tail regeneration. Nat Cell Biol 15: 222–228 (2013). doi: 10.1038/ncb2659

[19] Dvorak HF. Tumors: wounds that do not heal. Similarities between tumor stroma generation and wound healing. N Engl J Med 315(1986): 1650–1659. doi: 10.1056/NEJM198612253152606

12. MATHEMATICAL MODELS OF CANCER

12.1 Establishment of Cancer Development Model

Cancer immunoediting occurs in three sequential phases: elimination, equilibrium, and escape. As tumors progress, an increase in mutations may lead to the emergence of more immunologically inert cancer cells, which may upregulate the expression of immune checkpoint regulators through certain gene mutations or overexpression, thereby evading immune surveillance. Additionally, more subtle mechanisms involve the recruitment of actively immunosuppressive inflammatory cells, including regulatory T cells (Tregs) and myeloid-derived suppressor cells (MDSCs). Escape from immune control is now recognized as one of the hallmarks of cancer. Consequently, the tumor's immune clearance capability gradually diminishes, ultimately leading to the tumor breaking through immune equilibrium and escaping immune surveillance. In our 4T1 model, a declining trend in the immune system's ability to suppress cancer cells is also observed.

The immune system's capacity to kill and clear cancer cells should progressively decrease over time, potentially manifesting as a decreasing proportion of new cancer cells that can be killed by the immune system.

We hypothesize that within a time interval Δt, a proportion ρ of the new cancer cells are sensitive to the immune system, which can eliminate these cells. Conversely, a proportion $1-\rho$ of the cells are resistant to the immune system. Furthermore, ρ decreases over time t, defined by $\rho = \frac{\beta}{1+k_2 t}$, where β represents the initial immune clearance proportion at t=0.

The total number of cancer cells, V(t), continuously divides to generate new cancer cells. However, due to immune system clearance, a portion of the newly formed cancer cells will die. Therefore, we have:

$$\frac{dV}{dt} = k_1 V \left(1 - \frac{\beta}{1 + k_2 t}\right)$$

$$(S1)$$

Where k_1 represents the proportion of all newly added cancer cells.

Integrating equation (S1), we can obtain the tumor burden function represented by the total number of cancer cells:

$$V(t) = V_0 \frac{e^{k_1 t}}{(1 + k_2 t)^{\beta \frac{k_1}{k_2}}}$$

$$(S2)$$

The tumor burden index is equivalent to the total number of cancer cells: V(t); the immune clearance coefficient is β, which decreases over time according to the function $\frac{1}{1 + k_2 t}$. This model ensures: 1) Tumor occurrence follows an exponential pattern; 2) The immune system is influenced by the remaining tumor cells, with the absolute value continuously increasing. However, as the remaining tumor cells grow, the relative growth slows down, reflecting the dynamics of immune editing. This also aligns with the situation in the 4T1 model discussed in the preclinical research report in the previous chapter, where the immune enhancement in the treatment group does not exhibit long-lasting effects.

12.2 Estimating Model Parameters Using Preclinical Research Data

Since the tumor burden index growth rate in mouse cancer models far exceeds that in humans, we assume that one day in mice is equivalent to one month in humans. Furthermore, we assume that a clear signal of cancer occurrence appears at time t=0, with V(0) =1, and patient death occurs when the tumor burden index reaches 10. Based on our 4T1 model, the moment when the tumor volume reaches 4000mm3 in mice can be used to predict mouse mortality. In the untreated group, the tumor burden increases by a factor of 10 in approximately 17 days (from the 16th day to the 33rd day after 4T1 tumor implantation). Considering that cancer detection in humans often lags behind the earliest signals, we estimate that the tumor burden index for humans lies between 1 and 10. Following an exponential growth curve, we can roughly estimate this midpoint's tumor burden index to be 3.53.

Results from a clinical trial on advanced colorectal cancer (n=28) indicate that patients' average survival period after treatment with Panitumumab is 17.95 months. Taking into account late-stage factors and treatment effects offsetting each other, 17 months represent half of the overall cancer progression period for this group of cancer patients. Therefore, we assume that for a typical cancer patient, the tumor burden index increases from 1 to 10 in approximately 34 months, which is twice the duration in the mouse model.

Referring to fig, S1A, the exponential growth coefficient of the fitted line for the untreated mouse tumor burden curve is 0.15. Hence, we estimate that the growth coefficient for the tumor burden index in humans should be close to half of this value, around 0.75. Considering the impact of immune clearance capacity, we can roughly estimate that k_1 is slightly greater than 0.75. Since cancer cells are in an immune evasion phase, the value of

$$\frac{\beta}{1+k_2 t}$$

ranges from 0 to 0.25 and decreases approximately linearly. Taking all factors into account, we can roughly estimate: $k_1 = 0.08$; $k_2 = 0.02$; $\beta_1 = 0.2$.

12.3 Mathematical Models of Cancer Treatment

1. Treatment without Drug Resistance (Chlorine Dioxide Intra-Tumor Injection Model)

Since chlorine dioxide kills cancer cells through an oxidative chemical process, and our regenerative damage experiments have also shown that chlorine dioxide's cancer cell killing is non-selective, the variable of drug resistance is not reflected in this model.

From the function $V(t) = V_0 \dfrac{e^{k_1 t}}{(1+k_2 t)^{\beta \frac{k_1}{k_2}}} = \delta$, we can solve for $t = T(\beta, \delta)$. δ_1 represents the tumor burden index before treatment, and treatment is administered at time t_1 with CD intra-tumor injection. After treatment, the tumor burden index diminishes to $\alpha\delta_1$, where the tumor shrinkage rate α is directly related to the CD dosage—the higher the CD dosage, the greater the shrinkage rate. The cancer occurrence and immune clearance capacity return to time $t_{-1} = T(\beta_1, \alpha\delta_1)$. The time of death is when the tumor burden index reaches δ_2. Therefore: $t_1 = T(\beta_1, \delta_1)$; the expected survival period before treatment is $t_2 = T(\beta_1, \delta_2)$; due to treatment reducing the tumor burden index and the immune clearance capacity returning to the state at time t_{-1}, we express this as the tumor burden index function changing from V(t) to V(t-Δt) after treatment, with the parameter β changing from β_1 to β_2; $\Delta t = t_1 - t_{-1} = T(\beta_1, \delta_1) - T(\beta_1, \alpha\delta_1)$. After treatment, the new expected survival period is $t_{2n} - \Delta t = T(\beta_2, \delta_2)$, extending the survival period due to treatment:

$$t_{2n} - t_2 = T(\beta_2, \delta_2) - T(\beta_1, \delta_2) + T(\beta_1, \delta_1) - T(\beta_1, \alpha\delta_1) \qquad \text{(S3)}$$

Using CD treatment for cancer enhances immune capacity, indicated by $\beta_2 > \beta_1$, and $\frac{\partial T}{\partial \beta} > 0$, leading to $T(\beta_2, \delta_2) - T(\beta_1, \delta_2) > 0$. Since $\delta_1 > \alpha\delta_1$ and $\frac{\partial T}{\partial \delta} > 0$ we find that $T(\beta_1, \delta_1) - T(\beta_1, \alpha\delta_1) > 0$. The difference $T(\beta_2, \delta_2) - T(\beta_1, \delta_2)$ represents the contribution of enhanced immunity to the extension of survival time, while $T(\beta_1, \delta_1) - T(\beta_1, \alpha\delta_1)$ represents the contribution of tumor ablation to extending the survival period.

Using a treatment method that directly ablates tumors, the tumor burden index curve shifts backward (V(t) $\rightarrow$ V(t-n)), resembling a reversion to an earlier state in the cancer progression. This indicates a restoration of the immune system's capacity to clear cancer cells to the state at time (t-n), which is effectively an increase in clearing capacity. However, this does not imply an enhancement in immune function, but rather a relative advantage due to the reduced tumor burden. If such a treatment additionally boosts immune capacity, it would mean an increase from β_1 to β_2, resulting in a flatter tumor burden curve (Fig. S1A). In our 4T1 model, we can consider the control group of the small tumor cohort (PBS+ST) as an earlier stage (t-n) of tumor development compared to the control group of the large tumor cohort (PBS+LT), and the treated small tumor cohort (CD+ST) as an earlier stage (t-n_{treat}) of the treated large tumor cohort (CD+LT). We estimate β_2 to be 0.4, assuming that one day in mice corresponds to one month in humans.

Setting $t_0=0$ and $V_0=0$, and using Excel with the parameters above, we can generate the typical cancer progression curve and the curve showing intra-tumoral CD injection treatment (Figure A).

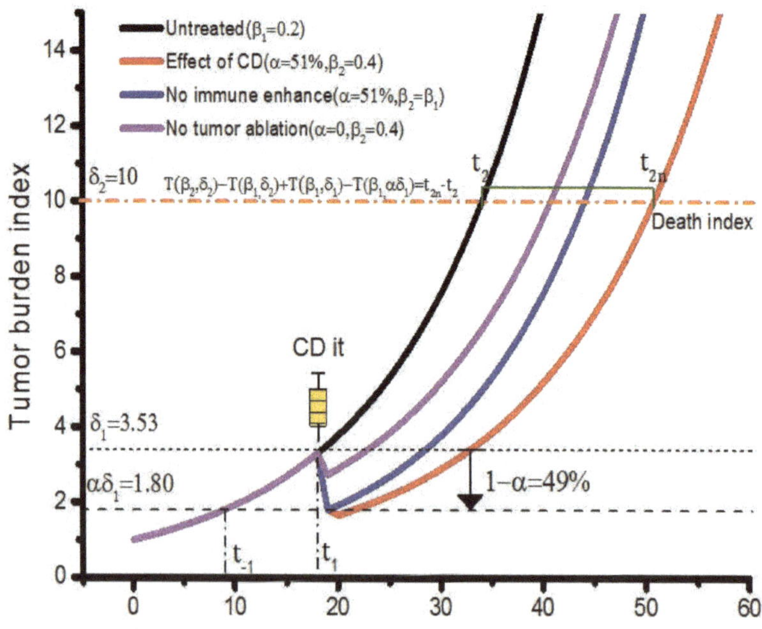

Figure A. Parameters are set as follows: β_1=0.2; k_1=0.08; k_2=0.02; and t represents time (days for mice, months for humans). A CD therapy is administered when the tumor burden index $\delta1$ reaches 3.53, with a mortality threshold at δ_2=10. This treatment method results in direct tumor reduction ($\alpha\delta$) and changes in immune capability (β_2=0.4). Consequently, when the tumor burden is reduced to 51% of its original size (α=51%), the entire tumor burden curve shifts to an earlier stage by several periods (t-Δt), equivalent to delaying the progression of the tumor burden curve by several periods (when 1-α=0.49, Δt=10).

When V(t) reaches $\delta1$ = 3.5, treatment with intra-tumoral CD injections begins. After treatment, the tumor burden decreases to $\alpha\delta\_1$, where $0 < \alpha < 1$. When the tumor burden index reaches $\delta2$, the patient is considered to have reached the end of life. Following treatment, the patient's survival period can be extended as:

$$t_{2n} - t_2 = T(\beta_2, \delta_2) - T(\beta_1, \delta_2) + T(\beta_1, \delta_1) - T(\beta_1, \alpha\delta_1)$$

$$(S3)$$

Using Excel to simulate calculations, increasing the tumor ablation ratio (1-α) and anti-tumor immune capacity ($\gamma\beta$) can extend the patient's survival period (see Fig. S1B-C).

We envision a method of using CD for periodic and intermittent tumor ablation. This approach starts intra-tumoral injection ablation treatment when the tumor burden reaches a clinically observable level. After CD ablates the tumor, it not only has a direct ablation effect but also does not cause drug resistance and can enhance immune capacity. This keeps the tumor burden within a safe range, transforming cancer with solid tumors into a true chronic condition where patients do not die from cancer (Figure. B).

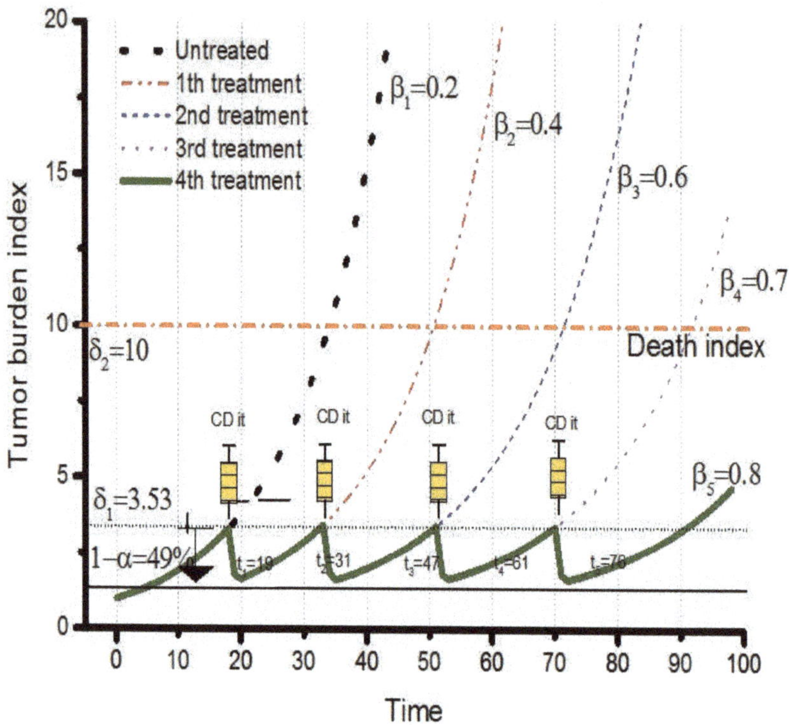

Figure. B Each ablation reduces the tumor burden (α=51%) and enhances immune capability, ensuring that the tumor burden curve never reaches the mortality line.

Traditional treatment approaches often focus on one aspect while neglecting another. However, combination therapies have shown better treatment outcomes (see Fig. S1D). Based on our experiments and mathematical models, we have learned that: 1) Tumor burden follows an exponential growth curve; 2) Immune surveillance is constant, but the growth rate of anti-tumor immune capabilities cannot keep up with the increase in cancer cells, leading to eventual immune escape by the cancer cells; 3) The goal of cancer treatment is to enhance both the anti-tumor immune response and the direct ablation of tumors, with direct ablation proving more efficient than boosting immune capabilities; 4) If tumors are ablated without enhancing immune capabilities, cancer cells will continue to grow along their original trajectory, and both tumor burden and anti-tumor immune capabilities will revert to their early states, possibly giving the immune system a relative advantage; 5) Intra-tumoral CD injections can easily ablate specific tumors (unaffected by cancer cell mutations and without inducing drug resistance), significantly delaying cancer progression, restoring the dominance of immune surveillance, and also provoking additional immune responses that exert pressure on distant and metastatic tumors.

2. Treatments Facing Drug Resistance: Chemotherapy and Targeted Drug Therapies

When cancer is clinically diagnosed, treatments that can lead to drug resistance, such as chemotherapy or targeted drug therapies, are often employed. The tumor burden is described by $V(t) = V_s + V_r$, where V_s and V_r represent the populations of drug-sensitive and drug-resistant cancer cells, respectively: $V_s = sV(t)$; $V_r = rV(t)$; $s + r = 1$.

Chemotherapy and targeted drugs typically kill only the sensitive cancer cells, having no effect on the resistant ones. After a period of treatment, these drugs can effectively halt the proliferation of the sensitive cells, reducing their growth rate to zero. The recurrence or progression of cancer is then solely dependent on the growth rate of the resistant cells. This is a key difference between resistant and non-resistant treatment methods.

Within the tumor, cancer cells compete for space and resources. Higher doses of chemotherapy or targeted drugs can kill a portion of the sensitive cells, reducing the overall tumor burden. However, due to the heterogeneity of the tumor, the resistant cells may actually proliferate faster due to the newly available space and resources left by the death of the sensitive cells. This results in a scenario where the more sensitive cells die off (the greater the value of $s - d_s$), the faster the remaining resistant cells grow. Here, d_s represents the proportion of sensitive cells remaining after treatment with chemotherapy or targeted drugs.

Due to ample living space and resource availability, the proliferation rate of drug-resistant cancer cells can be divided into two parts: one that continues at the original rate and another that accelerates due to the abundant supply of space and resources. This can be expressed as:

$$\frac{dV_r}{dt} = k_1 V_r \left(1 - \frac{\beta}{1 + k_2 t}\right) + k_3 \frac{(s - d_s)}{t} V_r$$

（S4）

k_3 represents the proportion of drug-resistant cells that increase due to the space and resources made available by the death of sensitive cancer cells. During treatment, d_s remains constant (assuming that after chemotherapy or targeted drug therapy, the total number of sensitive cancer cells decreases to a stable level, a process that occurs from t=0 to t=3), and is represented by $d_s = \alpha s$, where α is the residual proportion of sensitive cancer cells after anti-cancer treatment. Time is recalculated starting from t=3, implying that this treatment method increases the death of sensitive cancer cells, thereby enhancing immune clearance capabilities, which we simplify here to the immune clearance capabilities at t=3. We define $k_4 = k_3 \, (s - d_s)$. Integrating this can yield:

$$V_r(t) = V_{r0} \frac{e^{k_1 t} t^{k_4}}{(1 + k_2 t)^{\beta(\frac{k_1}{k_2})}}$$

（S5）

This leads to the development of a model for cancer progression under drug-resistant treatment::

$$V(t) = d_s V_0 + \; (1 - s) \; V_0 \frac{e^{k_1 t} t^{k_4}}{(1 + k_2 t)^{\beta(\frac{k_1}{k_2})}}$$

（S6）

Before treatment, the tumor burden function remains as (S2), with parameters k_1=0.08, k_2=0.02, and β_1=0.2. Since this is a treatment that can induce drug resistance, the model parameters are set as s=0.8 and k_3=0.8. Simulations conducted using Excel software result in Figure 4H. The simulation reveals that starting treatment with a drug that can cause resistance, the larger the dose, the more the tumor shrinks, but the less the expected survival time of the patient extends. If the drug dosage is reduced to just prevent the proliferation of sensitive cancer cells without reducing their number, the patient's expected survival time is longer. This finding aligns with the research by Pedro M. Enriquez-Navas and others.

Some forms of radiation therapy can also induce drug resistance. Although different doses of radiation therapy can extend survival, cancer recurrence is inevitable, and the relationship between different doses of radiation therapy and improved survival is complex. Our mathematical model can explain these complex relationships and is consistent with the results from Kevin Leder and others' Glioblastoma animal radiation therapy experiments and optimized mathematical models.

It is evident that cancer treatment becomes more complex with methods that induce drug resistance, and these methods do not necessarily prolong patient survival continuously. Based on this mathematical model of drug-resistant treatment, it's easy to conclude that increasing the proportion of sensitive cancer cells, s (for example, from 0.5 to 0.8), allows for further suppression of cancer cells and prolongs patient survival (Fig. S2). Therefore, compared to using a single dose of targeted drugs, a combination of multiple targeted drugs can significantly inhibit the growth of animal tumors or significantly extend patient survival. Our model also accurately predicts that low-dose, high-frequency metronomic chemotherapy alone or a combination of different types of drugs can offer greater benefits to patients, consistent with extensive clinical data.

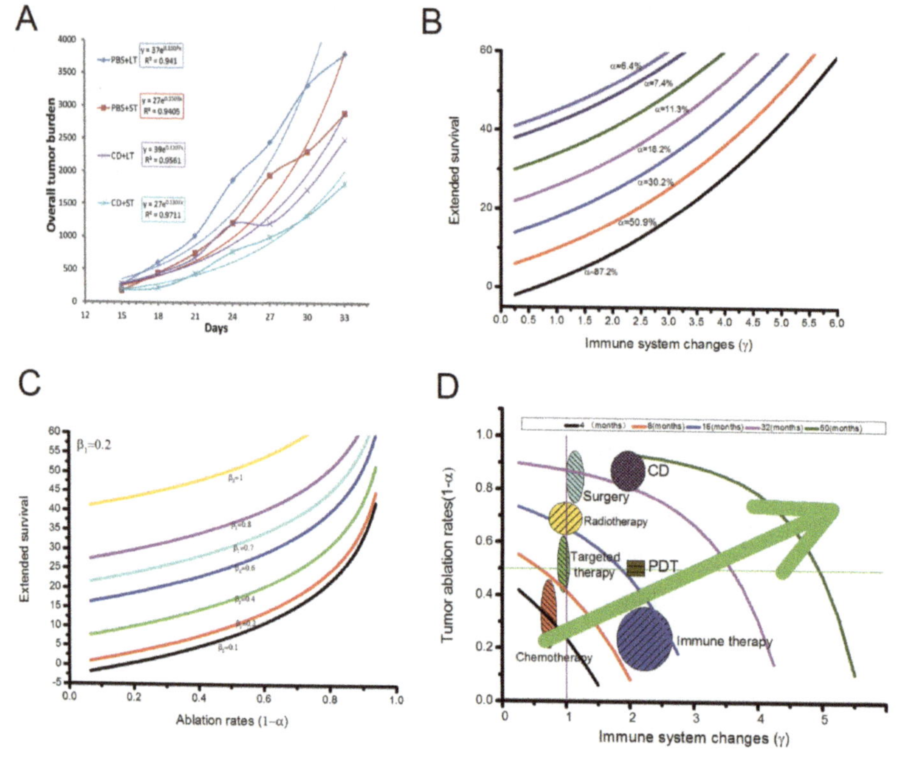

Fig. S1 The 4T1 tumor growth model and CD intratumoral injection treatment mathematically (A) In the study, we combined the volumes of axillary and mammary pad tumors to measure the total tumor burden in mice. We observed the growth curves for both large and small tumors. For large tumors, we analyzed the control group (PBS+LT) and the treatment group (CD+LT). Similarly, for small tumors, we examined the control group (PBS+ST) and the treatment group (CD+ST). Each group's tumor growth was fitted with an exponential curve using Excel. It's important to note that these calculations did not include tumors that metastasized to the lungs. If these metastatic tumors were considered, the overall tumor burden growth would align more closely with an exponential model. (B) In the CD intratumoral injection treatment model for cancer, factors affecting survival extension include an increased immune response. The relationship between increased immunity and extended survival is represented by the difference $F^{-1}(\beta_2, \delta_2) - F^{-1}(\beta_1, \delta_2)$, which increases logarithmically with β, where $\beta_2 = \gamma\beta_1$. (C) The relationship between tumor ablation proportion and survival extension, $F^{-1}(\beta_1, \delta_1) - F^{-1}(\beta_1, \alpha\delta_1)$, increases exponentially with 1-α. (D) The combined effect of tumor ablation proportion and increased immunity on extending survival highlights a critical decision in cancer treatment: whether to directly eliminate cancer cells or enhance immune cells to clear them. Ideally, enhancing both strategies is the optimal approach. Existing treatments offer various combinations of these methods, each affecting survival extension differently (targeted therapies and surgery impact only ablation; chemotherapy affects ablation but also damages immune capacity; radiation therapy affects ablation with a slight boost to immunity; immunotherapy primarily boosts immune capacity and suppresses tumors through this mechanism; PDT directly ablates tumors and triggers an anti-tumor immune response, though its ablation proportion is not high due to complex procedures and limited to superficial tumors; CD intratumoral injection can directly ablate tumors and potentially trigger an immune response, offering convenience in use). The strategic combination in cancer treatment should aim to expand the combined effects towards the upper right corner: increasing direct ablation proportion and enhancing anti-tumor immunity.

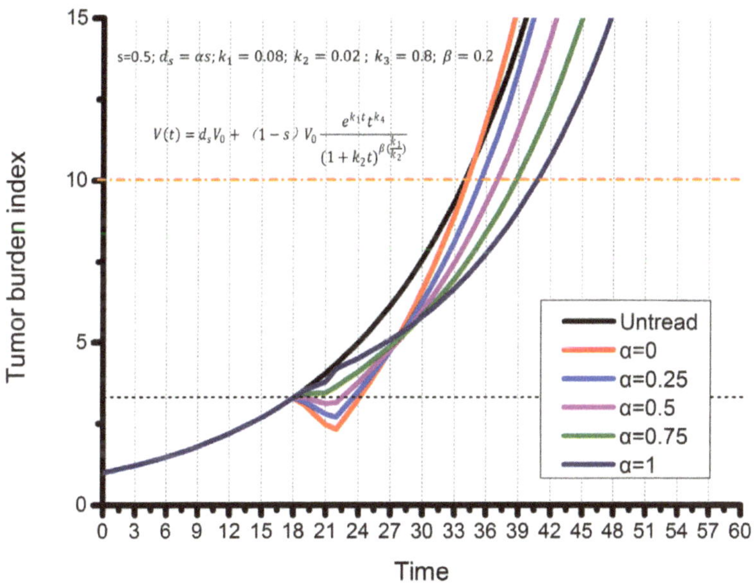

Fig. S2. Mathematical Model of Drug Treatment Resulting in Resistance.

V_0 represents the initial tumor burden index at the start of cancer treatment, is set at 3.3. When treatment begins with a drug that causes resistance, a higher dosage results in more significant tumor reduction but a shorter extension of the patient's expected survival. Conversely, reducing the drug dosage to a level that only maintains the non-proliferation of sensitive cancer cells without shrinking them results in a longer expected survival time. This model applies to a scenario where the proportion of drug-sensitive cancer cells is low, with (s = 0.5).

Additional References

1) Dunn GP, Bruce AT, Ikeda H, Old LJ, Schreiber RD. Cancer immunoediting: from immunosurveillance to tumor escape. Nat Immunol. 3:991–8(2002).
2) Hanahan D, Weinberg RA. Hallmarks of cancer: the next generation. Cell.144:646–74(2011).
3) Keisuke K, Yuichi S, Yohei T, Seiji S, et al. Aberrant PD-L1 expression through 3'-UTR disruption in multiple cancers. Nature. 1476-4687(2016).
4) Casey SC, Tong L, Li Y, Do R, Walz S, et al. MYC regulates the antitumor immune response through CD47 and PD-L1. Science. Apr 8;352(6282):227-31(2016).
5) Ostrand-Rosenberg, S., and Sinha, P. Myeloid-derived suppressor cells: linking inflammation and cancer. J. Immunol. 182, 4499–4506(2009).
6) Mougiakakos, D., Choudhury, A., Lladser, A., Kiessling, R., and Johansson, C.C. Regulatory T cells in cancer. Adv. Cancer Res. 107, 57–117(2010).
7) Jr, L. A. D., Williams, R., Wu, J., Kinde, I., Hecht, J. R., & Berlin, J., et al. The molecular evolution of acquired resistance to targeted egfr blockade in colorectal cancers. Nature, 486(7404), 537-40(2012).
8) Merlo, L. M., Pepper, J. W., Reid, B. J., & Maley, C. C. Cancer as an evolutionary and ecological process. Nature Reviews Cancer. 6(12), 924-35(2006).
9) R. A. Gatenby, R. J. Gillies, A microenvironmental model of carcinogenesis. Nat. Rev. Cancer. 8, 56–61 (2008).
10) Enriquez-Navas, P. M., Kam, Y., Das, T., Hassan, S., Silva, A., & Foroutan, P., et al. Exploiting evolutionary principles to prolong tumor control in preclinical models of breast cancer. Science Translational Medicine, 8.327 (2016).

11) Leder, K., Pitter, K., Laplant, Q., Hambardzumyan, D., Ross, B. D., & Chan, T. A., et al. Mathematical modeling of pdgf-driven glioblastoma reveals optimized radiation dosing schedules. Cell, 156(3), 603-16(2014).

12) Crystal AS, Shaw AT, Sequist LV, Friboulet L, Niederst MJ, Lockerman EL, et al. Patient-derived models of acquired resistance can identify effective drug combinations for cancer. Science. 346(6216):1480–1486. science.1254721(2014).

13) Ivana Bozic, Johannes G Reiter, Benjamin Allen, Tibor Antal, Krishnendu Chatterjee, Preya Shah, Yo Sup Moon, Amin Yaqubie, Nicole Kelly, Dung T Le, Evan J Lipson, Paul B Chapman, Luis A Diaz, Jr, Bert Vogelstein, Martin A Nowak. Evolutionary dynamics of cancer in response to targeted combination therapy. Elife, 2(12), 2260-2275 (2013).

14) André, N., Carré, M., & Pasquier, E. Metronomics: towards personalized chemotherapy?. Nature Reviews Clinical Oncology, 11(7), 413-31(2014).

ABOUT THE AUTHOR

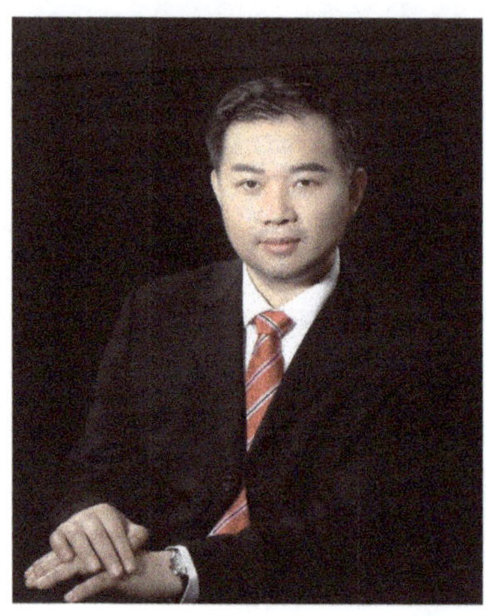

Xuewu Liu, a Chinese national, graduated from Nanjing University in 1998 with a Bachelor's degree in Atmospheric Physics and Atmospheric Environment from the Department of Atmospheric Science. He later obtained his Master's degree in Economics from the School of International Business at Nanjing University in 2001. Despite not having a background in biomedicine, Liu has a strong grasp of complex scientific concepts. Throughout his career, he has worked in government departments, financial institutions, and private investment firms, showcasing his profound scientific knowledge and innovative thinking in economics and business management.

The author has gained experience in three typical complex scientific fields and has developed a promising intratumoral injection drug. Through this process, he formulated an effective approach to solving complex scientific problems, which coincidentally aligns with the principles of first principles thinking. As a cross-disciplinary professional entering the field of cancer, the author deeply feels the plight of cancer treatment—a field dominated by overconfident doctors, presumptuous researchers, and traditionalist regulators, with hardly any satisfied cancer patients.